THE TRUTH ABOUT NURSING
Reflections of a Young Nurse

Rebecca Parker, MSN, RN, FNP-C
Copyright © 2017 Rebecca Parker

All rights reserved.

ISBN:1979046840
ISBN-13:9781979046848

Edited by Gabrielle Schoenrock

DEDICATION

To my loving parents, to whom I owe everything.
and
to my husband.

CONTENTS

Introduction
    i. What is Nursing Anyway?....................3
    ii. How to Know if Nursing is For You..........4
    iii. Getting into Nursing School................. 11
    iv. How to do Well in Your Pre-Requisites.....15
    v. The Truth About Your GPA....................26

Part I: A Typical BSN Program/Nursing School
    Chapter 1: The Classes and Content (With Stories, of Course)....................31
    Chapter 2: Surviving Nursing School..........103
    Chapter 3: The NCLEX........................115

Part II: On the Job
    Prologue....................................123
    Chapter 4: The CNA Experience..................126
        i. The Beginning..........................126
        ii. Creeper...............................133
        iii. Dementia.............................141
        iv. Wounds................................143
        v. Poop...................................144
        vi. Closing...............................145
    Chapter 5: Starting Out as an RN
        i. Pay....................................147
        ii. Med-Surge.............................149
        iii. Nursing Specialties...................151
        iv. Orientation..........................157
    Chapter 6: A Typical Day....................169
    Chapter 7: Shift Change.....................191
    Chapter 8: Charting.........................202
    Chapter 9: 12-Hour Shift Survival Tips.........220
    Chapter 10: Miscellaneous Stories.................226
        -PCA Pump Problem........................226

- Blood on the Floor................................233
- Chest Tubes......................................234
- PainFULL Patients and Other Lessons in
  Customer Service...............................241
- My Advice..252
- Shaved Head......................................256
- Munchausen Syndrome..............................257
- Grossest Thing...................................262
- Most Rewarding Case..............................263
- NG Tubes and Altered Mental Status...............264
- Dementia & Blood Draw............................268
- Sudden Death.....................................268
- Obituaries.......................................279
- Blessing...280
- Breast Cancer....................................281
- TLC Despite Rudeness.............................282
- The 14-Hour Day..................................285
- More Advice......................................298

Chapter 11: Dealing with Doctors....................300
Chapter 12: Charge Nurse............................324
Chapter 13: Final Closing...........................327
  i. Why Nursing is Great...........................327
  ii. Read..333
  iii. Your Invitation..............................337
APPENDIX..340

THE TRUTH ABOUT NURSING

INTRODUCTION

Odds are if you're reading this, you (or someone you know) is thinking about becoming a nurse. After all, it sounds like a noble profession, right? When I was a little kid, being a nurse was on the list of things I wanted to be when I grew up, along with doctor, scientist, veterinarian, writer, and missionary. I decided to write this book mainly to help people, and specifically, to help new nurses and those who want to be nurses. In my brief time as a registered nurse (RN), I've learned that there are a lot of misconceptions about the profession of nursing, which I'll elaborate on throughout this book. I'm eager to share my experiences with you. In the following pages, I'll discuss what exactly nursing is, the ins and outs of nursing school, as well as what else it takes to earn those two glorious letters behind your name. I'll share stories from my first two years of work as an RN. I'll describe in detail my experiences working with mean doctors as well as both difficult and inspiring patients. Some of my stories are scary. Some will make you laugh. Some are embarrassing. Some will make you cry. Some will make you think. I'll also address topics you've probably heard other nurses talk about and wondered about yourself: charting, death, old naked people, emergencies, and money. If you are an aspiring nurse or already a new nurse, thanks for picking up this book. I hope my stories will help you on your journey.

Before you dive in, please note a few things. At the time I finished writing this book, I had been an RN for a mere two years. I understand that one day I will look back at my life and laugh at how little I knew and probably be humiliated that I published this. As you read, keep in mind that at the time of writing, I was indeed a brand new nurse myself. Also, please note that I have worked *one* job as an RN and in just *one* hospital as an RN. Nursing school programs vary. Hospitals vary. Nursing units and floors vary. Nursing practices may be different from state to state and from country to country. Policies are different in different places. Management varies. Remember as you read that this is *my* story and these are *my* experiences and thoughts. I do try to lay out the facts for you as well but at times I do express personal opinion when we get into controversial topics (and real-life stories of course). If I offend you, feel free to stop reading but please do understand that if *I* offend you, you should probably not pursue a career in nursing. And yes, I have reassigned fake names to the real people and places in these stories in order to protect both the innocent and the not so innocent.

What is Nursing Anyway?

Before we start talking about nurses, nursing school, and nursing in general, it's fitting that we first define what exactly nursing is. Simply stated, and this is my definition here, **nursing is taking care of sick people**. This looks like a lot of different things. It's doing what a doctor says to do (some people would take offense to this). It's administering medications. It's bathing people. It's feeding people. It's monitoring vital signs. It's doing cardiopulmonary resuscitation (CPR). It's cleaning up poop. It's telling people (educating) about a diagnosis and how it's treated. It's working with doctors and physical therapists and other people on the health care team to help people achieve health and wellness. It's providing pain relief, whether that's with pain meds, heat, ice, etc. Nursing means providing care and help to someone who is sick or unable to care for themselves. It's nurturing. It's giving of yourself to help another person who is in need.

Rebecca Parker

How to Know if Nursing is for You

First let me say, don't go into nursing for the money. Yes, you can make a decent living in this role, but if that's your reason for pursuing nursing, you're going to hate your life. And people.

Beginning in 8th grade, I developed a really fond interest in the human body, and particularly in muscles, bones, ligaments, and tendons. Perhaps this was because I played sports. I suffered from a bad ankle sprain during basketball practice one day. Despite the pain and the frustration of having to sit out a week, I thought the way my body responded to the injury by swelling and turning my ankle black and blue was so cool. Eighth grade was also when I discovered weight lifting. I thought it was neat how over time the body could get stronger when exposed to stress. I loved health and PE class, and I loved sports. As I ventured through high school and began to think about college, I considered going into physical therapy. My academic advisor encouraged me to pursue occupational therapy since math and science weren't really deemed my strong suits.

I entered college believing physical therapy would be my niche. I quickly changed my mind after my mom had shoulder surgery and I attended one of her physical therapy sessions. The rehab gym was impressive, with huge plastic balls, dumbbells, ropes, and other fancy equipment used to restore function. I appreciated the physical therapist's desire to improve people's lives by restoring their mobility and independence, but I just couldn't visualize myself spending 40 hours a week in that gym. I also thought it would get old fast and that I'd master almost everything the field had to offer too quickly and find myself bored after a short time (sounds a little haughty, I know).

After one semester at a private and overpriced college, I transferred to a public university. I continued taking my general education requirements once I got there. I had not declared my major as a freshman student; the thought of that terrified me. I did know that I was interested in biology and exercise science, but I also thought a lot about life after college and my ability to land a job with my given degree. One day I discovered that my school had a nursing program, so I ventured into the health sciences building which housed the nursing program. I somehow ended up in the advisor's office where I met Sandy and Barbie, two people who really encouraged me throughout my time in undergraduate (undergrad) studies. They explained to me a little about the university's nursing program and its requirements. Sandy became my main academic advisor.

Nursing sounded to me like a worthwhile degree to get. I've always been what I call a realist, someone who is hopeful and positive, but who also bases decisions on facts and reality, rather than intuition or wishful thinking. I thought things through. I had always been interested in the human body, nutrition, and medicine. I spent a decent amount of time soul-searching and researching different professions that sounded interesting (keep in mind I was 19-years-old here). With a degree in exercise science, I could be a fitness instructor and work at a gym. With a biology degree I could apply for medical school but then there was a thought that my degree wouldn't amount to much if I didn't get in to medical school on my first attempt. I wanted to be able to make decent money right out of college with my bachelor's degree but also not feel stuck in one area and then have to go back for another bachelor's degree in something else within a few years. I also wanted to make my father proud and happy, since he was funding this whole endeavor. I pondered all of these things and talked to some different people, including fitness trainers, pre-med students, and other respectable adults in my life.

My second semester of undergrad while I was taking general education classes, I volunteered at a small hospital near my home. I experienced the flow of several different nursing floors during this time, but spent most of my eight hours a week on the oncology ward. I felt so cool getting to wear my blue polo shirt and "volunteer" badge and khakis when I went in to volunteer. Having that badge made me look and feel important even though I didn't know a thing.

I mostly shadowed Anne and Valerie, both RNs. I remember them hanging blood for transfusions, administering medications, and talking to patients. They were always busy with something. Looking back now, it's funny how little I knew then. I remember once asking Anne, who was an older nurse, "What do you do if you walk into a room and a patient is lying there dead (or seemingly dead)?" She responded, "You'd call a code." It was left at that, as she took off to her next task. I remember wondering what a code was. Ha. The more I worked with and observed Anne and Valerie, the more my fascination grew. I liked the way that they had autonomy and appeared in charge of things. They were confident and worked well together.

Volunteering allowed me to see a lot. I volunteered 100 hours at the hospital that semester. Anne and Valerie encouraged me, as did many of the nurse aides. My main tasks as a volunteer were giving cups of ice water to the patients, talking to patients, retrieving blood from the lab for transfusions (which I thought was pretty cool; and now looking back, I'm sure it saved the nurses a lot of time), and occasionally being lucky enough to get my hands on some old-fashioned patient charts—the paper ones. I got to see transfusions, doctors interact with patients at the bedside, and observe some physical and occupational therapy. Again, I respected their jobs, but I was more attracted to what the nurses were doing. They seemed like the healers. They seemed like the ones really running the show.

I decided before even choosing the nursing program that I'd like to have the option of pursuing a career as a physician assistant (PA) or a medical doctor (MD) upon leaving the university. This meant I'd have to "take the hard classes." I expressed this to Sandy and Barbie, who explained to me the courses I needed to take. I also wanted to get into the nursing program. My ultimate goal was to graduate with my bachelor's degree in nursing so that I could start working right after graduating from college. At the same time, I wanted to have taken all the classes necessary to apply to PA school and/or medical school and to have a high GPA (grade point average). Obtaining a bachelor of science in nursing (BSN) would allow me to check the boxes on what I wanted to get out of my time in undergrad. That summer, I set my sights on becoming a nurse. With the help of my advisors, I began taking the pre-requisite classes needed to apply for my school's nursing program (we'll talk about this soon).

I highly recommend volunteering to those of you thinking about becoming a nurse or going into the medical field. It has many benefits:

1) You're not a paid employee, so you can show up or not show up and leave when you want.

2) It looks great on a resume and can even open up a paid position for you.

3) It allows you to learn for free—I was like a sponge in the hospital, observing everything from different jobs of the workers to

patient fears to the color of scrubs and how they differentiated staff.

4) Volunteering allows you to work alongside people who are entrenched in the field you're considering going into. This gives you excellent insight into the pros and cons of the job.

5) It gets your mind off yourself, which is good for a lot of reasons. The bottom line is volunteer!

A lot of people think nursing is cool. And it is. But it is not for everybody. That's worth saying again. Nursing is *not* for everyone. There are good nurses and bad nurses and there are nurses that should've never become nurses, and then there are nurses that should have retired a long time ago because they're jaded, burned out, or bitter. It is a great career but it is also very challenging. You will earn every dime that's in your pay check (at least working day shift at my job). Seriously, don't become a nurse for the money. There are easier ways to make a living. If you think you'll never have another human's excrements in your hair, pause and reconsider this path. If you think you'll never have to scrub urine off the floor or clean vomit off your clothes, think again. If you think you'll be shielded from the obscenities of sexual harassment and verbal abuse, you're wrong. Oh, and if you like Thanksgiving, Christmas, other major holidays, nights, and weekends off, don't go into nursing.

In this line of work, you will see sorrow, heartbreak, evil, death, greed, disease, poverty, suffering, abuse, neglect, hate, and injustice (did I leave any out?). But you will also see and get to take part in joy, healing, reconciliation, goodness, life, selflessness, health, alleviation, caring, and love. If you're looking for a job or career that's easy and one in which you don't have to do much, nursing is not for you. If you're lazy or don't like people, are easily annoyed, impatient, or selfish, don't go into nursing. But if you like to serve others, comfort others, and give, read on. If you like to think and work with your hands, and help people, keep reading. If you find life in meeting the needs of others and if you want more than the typical 9-5 job; if you believe that you're here for a purpose, nursing might be for you.

Getting into Nursing School

Before I could even apply to my nursing program, I had to take a few pre-requisite courses. To my knowledge, all nursing programs require you to have had statistics (stats), sociology, anatomy and physiology (A & P), and basic chemistry (chem). Keep in mind too, that you need to have done well in these courses (see your specific school program's requirements). A & P is one class you'll really want to do well in because it will help you down the road in nursing assessment and critical care. The material will not go away once you finish the course.

Note that there are different types of nursing schools as well. Some schools offer licensed practical nurse (LPN) education, some offer associate degrees for registered nurses, and some offer bachelor's degrees for registered nurses. Licensed practical nurses are different from registered nurses. Registered nurses go to school longer, have more autonomy and responsibility than LPNs, and thus make more money than LPNs. Also note that LPNs typically are employed by doctor's offices, clinics, and nursing homes, whereas RNs are more likely to be found in the hospital setting. Also, nurses who work in management are the ones who have at least a bachelor's degree. LPNs and RNs with associate degrees do not. Of course, obtaining a BSN takes the longest.

Nowadays there are a lot of programs out there called "bridge programs." These allow LPNs to become RNs through more schooling. There are also programs that provide associate to bachelor's degree education. Today there are a lot of online nursing programs popping up too. I encourage everyone thinking about nursing to go straight for their bachelor's in nursing for several reasons:

1) It's usually best to knock it out in one period of time. No one likes going back to school, especially once they've started working. When you go straight for the BSN, you don't have to go from LPN to RN and then from RN to BSN. It's just more streamlined.

2) There is more of a demand from employers for nurses with their BSNs. As hospitals try to reach magnet status (a special recognition for hospitals; 80% of employed RNs at that facility must have their BSN), the BSN is becoming more of the gold standard for entry-level education for nurses.

3) If you decide after a few years of nursing that you want to go into management, administration, education, or advanced practice, guess what? You have to have your bachelor's degree before you can climb the corporate ladder or even go back to graduate school for advanced practice.

4) Do it while you're young. If your parents are willing to pay for your college education, take advantage of that while you're at the traditional 4-year university.

5) It saves you time and money in the long run.

6) A lot of these frequently-advertised LPN or even associate degree RN programs online are scam schools. They charge $40,000 for an associate degree when you could just get your BSN at a public university for the same price.

7) You'll make more money with your BSN.

8) The BSN gives you more flexibility in terms of places you can work.

Keep in mind that there are a lot of different nursing schools out there. Tuition costs vary accordingly. I recommend public universities for BSN programs. In the long run, they usually are the cheapest. If you can't afford a university, I would recommend a local community college for an associate degree in nursing. Clinically speaking, with your associate degree you can do essentially the same things as a nurse with a BSN. Just remember that you will eventually have to go back for that BSN at some point if you want to advance. In my opinion, pursuing a degree as an LPN is a waste of time. It's outdated, and you'll be very limited in your practice as a nurse. So go for that BSN!

Once you've decided what program you want to apply for, you'll have to look at the admissions criteria for that particular program. Make sure you've taken the required pre-requisite (pre-req) courses, or else your application won't even be considered. I'm sure some nursing programs require an essay, letters of recommendation, and maybe even an aptitude test. Some, like my university's program, only care about your grade point average (GPA). My university's program offered admission to the applicants with the highest GPAs (assuming pre-reqs were completed).

Like most things in life, getting into a competitive program or obtaining whatever it is that you want is the easy part. Staying in that program or keeping what you worked hard for is another story.

How to Do Well in Your Pre-Requisites

Sandy, my advisor, had convinced me to take Chemistry 115 that summer in order to be able to take A & P in the fall. Nursing majors at my school were only required to take Chem 101 and 102 (very basic chemistry) as pre-requisites into the program, but I chose to take the more challenging 115 course because it would also count as a pre-req toward medical school and physician assistant school (essentially killing two or three birds with one stone). Please take my advice on this, if you're not one who likes to cram and "just get by" in your courses, which I frown upon for anyone going into the health professions, you want to avoid taking summer courses because they squeeze 16 weeks of material into eight weeks. The summer I took Chem 115, I was spending four or five days a week in lectures and lab and then every other waking moment studying what we'd gone over in class. I put probably 50 hours a week into that course. I got a 64 on the first exam, a huge blow to someone used to consistently scoring in the 90s. After that first exam, I realized it was a bad idea to continue, as Chem 116 builds upon everything learned in 115. And those courses crammed 16 weeks of material into eight weeks.

I withdrew from Chem 115 about two weeks in. It simply showed up as a "W" on my transcript, which I thought would look repugnant to any admissions board, but figured it looked better than a C or an F and still not ever understanding anything that was "taught" in the course.

When it comes to being "taught" as an undergraduate student, I advise you to not set your hopes high. You will need to give a lot of yourself to undergraduate and pre-requisite courses. Learn something important now: The majority of your college professors, regardless of what RateMyProfessor.com (if that's even still around?) and university awards say about them, are *not* going to teach you. I don't say this in arrogance, but anything I learned in undergrad (for the most part), I taught myself. If I had relied on just sitting in a few 50 minutes lectures each week, I would have failed miserably. Granted, I didn't work during much of undergrad. Studying was my job. And I treated it like that. I read before and after each class, outlined chapters, printed off powerpoint lectures and filled in the blanks. If there was something I didn't get, I'd go to the tutoring center and hunt down the serious kids, those who I knew were headed for medical school or NASA. I'd have them explain things to me. And then when I thought I got it, I'd teach it to some other kid. If you can teach it, you know it. My point is, learning takes time. And if you want to be great at what you do, which I'm sure you do, take the time to learn. It's worth it. And the people you serve in your profession will be grateful for it. Be prepared to sacrifice your social life, sleep, and the feeling that you're missing out when everyone else is having a good time and you're stuck in the library studying.

So, in your classes, get after it (my basketball coach in high school used to tell us in pre-game pep talks— "Get after it!"). Pursue knowledge and understanding so you can have a solid foundation for clinical practice. Work hard. It will not (or at least should not) be handed to you. Obtain your nursing degree because you earned it.

Proverbs 25:1 - "It's the glory of God to conceal a matter. It is the glory of kings to search out a matter."

Proverbs 22:29 – "Do you see a man skilled in his work? He will stand in the presence of kings. He will not stand in the presence of unknown men."

Needless to say, I gave up on rushing my way out of undergrad. I took Chem 115 in the fall after withdrawing from it in the summer semester. On the first exam, I got a 112 (out of 100) and finished with an A in the course. I sought out every extra credit point. I spent hours practicing those "limiting reagent" questions. I did sample questions ad nauseam. If I couldn't find the correct answer in feedback immediately after answering the question, I didn't waste my time on it. I needed to know right after working the problem whether it was correct. This is a big part of how I learn.

Know how you learn. Do you learn by listening to lectures or by reading books? Do you learn more by studying alone or in a group? Do you benefit by reading in advance? Do you need to get your hands on things in order to understand? There's some good books out there with quizzes in them to help you determine your preferred learning style if you don't know. It's worth the few minutes to fill one out. Apply it. It will help you be efficient in your studies.

When I took A & P, which, by the way was my most eagerly anticipated class to take, Dr. Stern had each of us fill out one of those quizzes in a book so that we'd each be aware of how we learn. God bless the man, he wanted us to be successful and he sure enjoyed A & P, but he was by no means a good "teacher" in my opinion. A lot of his 50-minute lectures were spent mostly talking about how stupid Republicans are. One day I just walked out of class. Nonetheless, I took the learning quiz, and was essentially reminded of what I already knew—I need to know as I learn and do practice problems whether or not I am on the right track. I need feedback. Also, I benefit from taking notes while I read and learn; I need to study in a quiet place; and I prefer to study alone.

I happened to bump into Kate early on in Sterns' class. She too got the same results from the "how you learn test." We both preferred to study alone. BUT, Stern emphasized repeatedly and early on in his class that in order to succeed in his class, you had to get into a study group. A study group consisted of three to five people who studied the material in depth together. Stern said this was the only way to get an A in his class. I listened to the man's advice and teamed up with Kate and a few others. We started off the semester strong. We'd split up the chapters that were assigned for reading. Each person would pick two and become an expert in that material and then teach it to the rest of the group. We'd quiz each other on the names of bones and the functions of hormones, etc. That's how we learned.

I got a 64 on the first exam. This may seem like a shocker to one who is unfamiliar with Sterns' anatomy exams. Understand, however, that his exams were extremely difficult and he threw in a roughly 30-point curve automatically on each one. So essentially, scoring in the 60s was really like scoring in the 90s. I was happy about this. The thing that made Sterns' exams so hard was that we took them in the computer lab and the questions were administered by a test bank. Each exam got harder because the test bank got bigger. It was possible to get some of the same questions on two different exams. This is one reason study groups were great. Stern let us write down during each exam roughly five questions that we were unsure of and then take it back to our study group for discussion. If each one had five questions, there was a nice little chunk of the test bank that we had the key to. Also, I firmly believe that talking something through out loud really helps you to understand it. If you can say it and teach it to somebody, you know it.

    My advice: If you do prefer studying in a group, pick your study buddies wisely. One of the main reasons I've never been big on group study is because very little of the allotted study time is actually spent talking about A & P or whatever the group is supposed to be studying. People in a group tend to get off topic way too easily. But if you and your group can stay on topic, it can be a very good thing for learning.

When it comes to study buddies, there's some people you simply just want to avoid. I remember a couple days before the A & P final lab practicum. Kate and I and a handful of the devoted few had been practically living in that lab the whole semester. I'll never forget when one buffoon waddled up to me in the lab and asked, "What's this?," pointing to the pancreas model. I was dumbfounded. Let's just say he was one of the few of my colleagues who did not go on to become a doctor. Don't waste your time teaching people who don't want to learn or who simply want to use you so they can have the easy way out. Also look out for cheaters.

I've never considered myself to be that "naturally smart" person who can understand things and get by without much effort. I've always studied and put a lot of time into learning. And I've never been a procrastinator. In fact, my final year of undergrad, I'd often turn in papers a month or more in advance. In between clinicals, classes, wedding planning, church, and everything else, I used my time wisely. At the start of each semester, I encourage you to print off the syllabus for each class. Highlight test days and record everything in a planner. Being organized will save you a lot of problems. I did learn, however, that it can almost be disadvantageous for you to turn work in too early. If you don't document somewhere that you did turn an assignment in, you'll wonder the day before it's due whether or not you already finished it. Make notes to yourself. Life is busy, especially in nursing school, so plan ahead. Use your time wisely.

Find a good place to do your work, and work when you're at your best. Ideally, I preferred my desk at home in my room. I had a bathroom a few feet away, a refrigerator a few more feet away, water, a comfy (but not too comfy) chair, internet access, all of my books within reach, and a printer. Also, at home, I could wear whatever I wanted and have the room at the perfect temperature. It was best when I was home alone. Sometimes, though, home can be distracting. Dogs bark. Neighbors knock on the door. Family members don't always use their inside voices. Phones ring. So, I started retreating to Starbucks. Senior year, this became a place where I could be extremely productive. Somehow, the background music didn't distract me. It would often be very cold inside, but I made arrangements to deal with it. And somehow iced coffee helped to get me in "the zone." The neighborhood and school libraries were not the best places to study either because I wasn't allowed to eat there, the bathrooms were far away, or an occasional crazy person or screaming child would cause distractions. Figure out where you can get your work done. Have a place of productivity.

Another perhaps equally important key to studying efficiently and to being successful in nursing school (and perhaps in life in general), is learning to say no. Nursing students tend to be type-A, overachieving, help everyone all the time, deny yourself, be the best at everything all the time kind of people. Take my advice and do yourself a favor. Learn to say no. And better yet, learn to say no and not feel bad about it. It is so easy to become overcommitted while you're in school. There's a plethora of activities to fill your schedule with—church stuff, school clubs, work, volunteer stuff, exercise classes, and more. Know what is important to you and make that a priority. Just do know that if you choose to go to nursing school, it will demand a lot of time. Make school a priority if school is what you choose to do. Then allot time for family, friends, work, and extracurricular activities. Schedule your time outside of your studies so that you don't feel guilty. Just don't fill your plate to the point where school starts to suffer. Treat your schoolwork like a job.

I learned this lesson early on in college. It was six weeks into my freshman year and basketball tryouts were the next day. I had so much anxiety because I realized college basketball was much different than it was in high school. All my high school buddies knew I was at a particular school to play basketball because I was just that good. I tried talking myself into just playing through the first year. The more I thought about how sore my body constantly was, how little I really cared for my teammates, and how I wasn't going to go pro upon graduating, playing through the first year seemed like less and less of a sensible option in the grand scheme of my life. I explained all of this to one of my closest friends (who later became my husband). He simply told me, "Drop that crap." The very next day, I did. I quit basketball and transferred to another school once that semester was over. I finished with a 4.0 GPA. I got to spend more time studying, working out when I wanted to, and simply being happy that first semester. Never once have I regretted my decision to quit basketball. Things would be totally different if I had stayed at that initial private school...I'd be overwhelmed by debt, probably be making less money with a less exciting job, and probably have taken much longer to discover nursing.

The Truth About Your GPA

I became a self-made perfectionist at age 12. Now, many years down the road, I can confidently say that I have broken free, but not entirely, of perfectionism. I carried my straight A, must-excel-at-everything mindset all the way through my first year of college. Then in my second year, when I took statistics, I got an A-. Shriek! My GPA dropped from a glorious 4.0 to a shameful 3.97. I felt imperfect. This bothered me for a long time and I even contacted the professor to ensure that he had calculated my grade correctly. My instructor had originally said in his class that he didn't give pluses and minuses. When I asked him then, why I got an A – in his class, he said that my cumulative average grade at the end of the semester was borderline A/B and he figured it would benefit me to get an A – rather than a B+. I thanked him.

I proceeded, recovering the following semester with all As

once again. I wormed my way through chemistry, genetics, biology, organic chemistry, public speaking, and English with As. My first official B came my second semester of nursing school in gerontology (the study of the elderly) and I was quite upset over it. My actual grade was a 92.4 at the end of the semester, a mere tenth of a point away from an "A." I pointed this out to the teacher, who was not at all sympathetic. What was worse, that 0.1 point was the difference between an A and a B, not an A- and a B+, because they don't do that in the nursing program. So I was hit with a B. And as frustrating, irritating, annoying, and shameful as it was, I honestly believe that it was one of the best things that ever could have happened to me. I was no longer "perfect."

Although I no longer carried a 4.0 GPA, I still worked very hard in school. From that semester on, though, I believe I got at least one B. What made the nursing program "harder" was that the overall grade in the class was almost entirely based on three exams over the course of the semester. And each exam was about 50 questions, which meant I could only miss three out of 50 and still come out with an A. I was good at this in pharmacology, nursing theory, and nursing research, mainly because these were subject areas that only required memorizing facts. Tests that required me to think were much harder, but I almost liked them more than the fundamental fact-based exams. Nonetheless, it's very difficult to get an A in nursing school because of the grading scale. There are no pluses or minuses and to get an A, students must have a 93. In other undergrad courses outside of nursing, anything 90 or above would earn them at least an A-. A 92.5 or higher would mean a solid A. And then there was the B +, which was kinder to the GPA than a B. So, in nursing school, be prepared for your GPA to take a hit. Also note that in my nursing program (and I believe this goes for most nursing programs) anything below an 80 is failing.

I don't mean to intimidate perfectionists. I do want to tell you not to kill yourself. Looking back now, I wonder if I had been more of a straight B or even straight C student if I'd be in the same place I'm in right now. Probably not. With a 3.0 GPA, I probably would not have been admitted to one of the state's most competitive nursing programs, and I certainly would not have gotten in with a 2.0. When I applied to the nursing program, I was confident I'd get in, because all the admissions board looked at was GPA. I had that 3.97 at the time I applied. So yes, you should work very hard in those pre-nursing classes. Build up your GPA so that you can be one of those 400 applicants that gets one of the 50 seats. And yes, having a good GPA is important for graduate school. That's really the main reason it counts. Potential employers won't ask you during a job interview what your GPA was in undergrad. What I do want to point out is that you shouldn't get lost in getting a grade. Enjoy school. Learn because you like it and you want to learn. Do not neglect time on the weekend with your loved ones because you have a test on Monday or pass up a late-night phone conversation with the man you love because you have to get mentally prepared for a presentation in the morning. Balance and prioritization. They are the keys to success and happiness throughout school. And it's something you sort of have to figure out for yourself. Know what matters to you and make time for it.

Summary

Take all of what I said into consideration. Are you willing to work hard in school? Are you willing to sacrifice? Are you interested in the human body? Do you like to help people? Do you like to serve people? Have you talked to nurses? Have you tried working as a nurse aide/nursing assistant? Have you even volunteered in a hospital on a nursing floor? Just because Grey's Anatomy or "ER" is your favorite show it doesn't mean you should automatically go for a career in nursing. Believe me when I say, most doctors in the real world don't look like Patrick Dempsey and John Stamos. There's no such thing as locker room romance; you're lucky if you have time to go to the bathroom when you work in the hospital. Oh, and high heels and fancy attire don't really function well when you walk six miles a day at work and get vomit on your clothes. Get a realistic idea of what nursing is like by volunteering, researching, talking to nurses, and maybe becoming a nurse aide first before you wholeheartedly dive in. Believe me, the world doesn't need more indifferent nurses.

PART 1: A Typical BSN Program / Nursing School

Chapter 1: The Classes and Content (with Stories, of Course)

I've included an outline of the nursing school curriculum I went through so you can see the way it's really set up. I'll discuss here in depth the ins and outs of each course in nursing school. I've also inserted a lot of personal opinion about my experience. Please note that my academic load through nursing school might be a little bit different because I didn't know for sure right out of high school that I wanted to go into nursing. If you start out at a four-year university knowing that nursing will be your major, your academic track might be a little more streamlined than mine was. I took a lot of "extra" classes that you probably won't have to take.

I've also included in the APPENDIX of this book a lot of

papers I wrote in nursing school. I've included a lot of assignments so that you can get a feel for how much time this major requires. You can see for yourself how extensive some of your projects will be.

The first year of the program, we took Health Assessment I (with lab), Intro to Nursing Theory & Concepts, and Therapeutic Diets I (Nutrition-part I). This was just six credit hours of nursing classes. I also took Genetics that fall, for a total of nine credits. So yes, I was a part-time student then.

Health Assessment I. In my opinion, this is the most fun and probably most important class taken during nursing school. This class is a good reason why you should learn your A & P really well before you start nursing school. It will make nursing assessment so much easier. I became an expert in the lab (or hands-on) portion of this class. Each week, we learned a different system of the body, how to assess it, and I would read the pertinent textbook chapters several times. In the classroom on Mondays, Mrs. H would read the powerpoint slides to us on that particular system (Note: She did not teach, she just read what was on the screen—again reiterating my point that you must be committed to learning and to teaching yourself). Then on Friday mornings we'd go to the lab and practice assessing one another. Our homework consisted of properly documenting the assessment. The first thing we learned in lab was how to ask all of the appropriate health assessment questions. Basically, it was like interviewing someone and finding out her whole life story.

I was fortunate to randomly pair up with a good lab partner. She had gotten married just a few months prior to the start of the program and just learned she was pregnant. That first week, we took turns asking each other all of the questions—allergies, current medications, chronic illnesses, family history, social history, education history, and the like. It was super in depth. Let me just say that now that I am working as a staff nurse in the hospital, I know for a fact that you will not do any of this in-depth analysis of your patients, at least not on a cardiac/medical floor, unless you're doing the patient's admission paperwork. There simply isn't time for it. We focus on the major issues. But the health history is a good thing to learn. It is important to know as much about your patients as possible. Everything, whether big or small, affects a person's health in some way. I guess this was what our instructors wanted us to understand from the start.

In Health Assessment I, you learn where to put your stethoscope so you can hear the heart properly. You learn how to percuss (which you'll never do in the real world as an RN), to palpate (touch) correctly, and assess every other thing. It's good stuff to know. Now that I'm finally a real RN, the first thing I do each morning to start my shift is assess my patients. You can read their chart and know their history, but you've got to get in the room and get that baseline assessment first thing each morning. Know what their sensory deficits are; their mental status; what their mouths look like; what their lungs and heart sound like; what their skin looks and feels like; whether or not they're peeing and pooping; what their appetite's like, whether or not they can walk, if they have any peripheral vascular compromise, and whether it's from congestive heart failure (CHF), diabetes, or peripheral vascular disease (PVD). In order to know if something has changed in any way, for better or for worse, you must have some knowledge of what the baseline was. It is easy as an RN to just get into the routine of things and to sort of do a "going through the motions" assessment. Beware of this. Really assess your patients and think while you assess them so that you won't look like an idiot when the doctor asks you a question that you as the primary nurse for the patient should know the answer to.

As a nurse, I encourage you to take the time in school to learn how to properly assess your patients. Know what's normal and what's not. Learn the systems of the body. Assessment is so important in the real world of nursing. It's one of your major job responsibilities. If a patient begins to go south, it's on you 1) to recognize it 2) to intervene quickly and appropriately, and 3) notify the doctor if necessary. General assessment is easy. Just look at your patient the way you'd look at a stranger in the grocery store. Notice his or her shape and build. Is the person overweight, underweight, or normal? Notice the person's facial expression and general appearance. Does he or she appear anxious or sad? Is he or she a little "odd"? Gather as much data as possible just by looking and listening and even smelling. Then go deeper. Whip out your pen light, stethoscope, and hands. Listen, see, measure, feel, smell. Don't worry about the taste aspect; I fortunately haven't had to use that one yet. Gather your data.

Intro to Nursing Theories and Concepts. If you're going to pick a class to fall asleep in, this is a good choice. I did have a very kind and knowledgeable instructor for this class, but at the time of taking the course I didn't see why it was necessary to spend two semesters learning about nursing theory. Nursing theory is basically just some other nurse's idea of what nursing is. We studied Florence Nightingale, Virginia Henderson, Orlando, and some of the other big name nurses and what their thoughts were on what nursing is and how it should be defined. Nursing theory is subjective, so again, to me it didn't make sense why it was so important to learn. I think the time spent in this class would have been much better spent in the clinical setting, but judge for yourself.

Please note: At the time of revising/editing this book, I have completed another nursing theory course, this time, at the graduate level. I've learned that nursing theory helps to define the profession of nursing, in much the same way that doctors have a defined set of standards that they practice by as well as the Hippocratic oath and other ethical principles that guide the doctor's actions. Theory helps to define a profession. I still don't think there's a need to spend two semesters learning about it, though.

One thing we did do in this class that was of great importance was write a paper on our own personal philosophy of nursing. Our instructor asked us to state how we define nursing and what the role of the nurse is. We had to explain the nurse's goals and assumptions. This paper was my favorite in all of undergrad to write because I really got to express myself and speak from the heart about a topic I was interested in. It was also a good idea for our instructor to have us write out a personal philosophy of nursing because it made us think about the profession and why we chose it.

We wrote this paper the first semester of the nursing program and then again in the final semester of the program. It was neat to compare the two. I have attached both papers for you to read (see Appendix). Whether your school requires you to write such a paper or not, I encourage nurses-to-be to engage in this exercise. I can tell you that just about three months into my career as a nurse, I had to pull this paper out a couple of times and remind myself of why I wanted to be a nurse. Believe me, you'll have your share of days (especially in the beginning) where you question if you've made the right career choice. This paper will be a good reminder to you of why you chose nursing and it will lift your spirit when the going gets rough.

Therapeutic Diets I. This is another easy class. A lot of the material covered is stuff you'll have already learned in Biology or A&P; or if you pay attention to what you eat half the time, this material will be easily understandable for you. The thing that made this class hard was that the grade was determined by just three multiple choice exams, each of which had 50 questions. There were no written papers that helped to make up the final grade. You can do fine in this course just with sheer memorization, but as always, actually learning the stuff and understanding it would be to your benefit.

Let's move on to the second semester of nursing school.

Intro to Nursing Theories part II. Again, this course was similar to the first half of Nursing Theory. I'm getting bored and distracted just thinking about this class.

Fundamentals of Nursing Practice. This is where we learned more about simple nursing skills like giving a bath, inserting catheters, using the bladder scanner, and making a bed (and yes, there is an art to that). It was basically a review of my certified nurse aide (CNA) course, which again, is why it's a good idea to consider being a CNA before you go into full-fledged nursing. The last six weeks of this course we got to spend in the hospital for a clinical rotation. This is where everybody got nervous because they'd actually have to interact with a real patient. Again, I was comfortable because of my CNA experience.

Students were divided into groups so that each clinical instructor would get about six or eight students. I was lucky enough to have Mrs. B as my clinical instructor. She was a spunky lady and laid-back compared to other instructors. She liked her job and didn't let it stress her out. She was also hands-off for the most part. We did our rotation on a basic medical floor. We got to see the typical things in older patients—renal failure, dementia, hypertension. During this first rotation, all we did was CNA-type work. We took vital signs, bathed and changed incontinent patients, and observed diagnostic tests like swallow studies and x-rays. It's funny to look back at. Yes, in addition to all of the cool and complex stuff you'll learn as a nurse, you will be responsible for all those simple, less glamorous tasks as well.

Please note that this is the semester that we were introduced to the dreaded care plan. In theory class, we were taught about the care plan, which outlined the nursing process: assessment, diagnosis, planning, implementation, and evaluation. Each week in clinical, we'd put this into practice. On Wednesdays, the day before we met our patients, we'd go to the hospital on our own time to get our patient assignment. We'd have to spend time looking at the patient's medical record and learning about them. Based on the patient's medical diagnosis, we'd have to compose a nursing diagnosis. Here's where medicine and nursing are different. I was taught that doctors treat illnesses and nurses treat the patient's response to the illness. This can mean a number of things.

 Imagine you're caring for a patient with stage 4 renal (kidney) failure. You, as the nurse, would then treat the effects that renal failure can have on the skin—itching, or rather, "skin breakdown." Or you could treat the effects of abnormal blood pressure (whether high or low)—safety concerns such as falling or "risk for falling." Nurses also treat anxiety or hopelessness, which can result from any chronic disease. There's a plethora of nursing diagnoses.

I've also been told that doctors treat diseases and nurses treat people. Please note that I am not hating on doctors. However, it is true that if you don't like people, you should not go into nursing. If you think you like people, nursing just might change your mind. You will see people at their worst and you will be the one who's expected to do something about it. Anyhow, do take the time to learn how to do these care plans properly because you will be expected to use them throughout the rest of your program. Will you use them as a real nurse? No. At least not exactly. But to become a nurse, you have to use them, so learn them. As a real nurse, you'll never write out the patient's nursing diagnosis or all of your in-depth assessment info, your interventions, or what the patient's response to it was (evaluation). You'll quickly learn that in the real world, there's just not time for that. The care plan in nursing school does prepare you to think like a nurse, though.

Pharmacology I (Pharm). This is a fun class. As a nurse, one of your main responsibilities will be to safely administer medications. In Pharm I you'll learn all about the drugs used to treat all kinds of illnesses (or responses to illnesses) that you as a nurse will encounter. You'll explore all the different classes of antihypertensive medications (blood pressure drugs), antiretrovirals (drugs that fight viruses), antibiotics (drugs that fight infection), antipsychotics (drugs that treat bipolar, schizophrenia, anxiety, etc.), analgesics (pain medications), and others.

A word to the wise: Don't get all wrapped up in and stressed out about memorizing which drugs are in which classes. They're not going to ask you that on the NCLEX. I know my Pharm teacher didn't test us on it. Some of the major blood pressures pills are good to know a lot about. It is important to know if metoprolol is going to lower your patient's blood pressure or heart rate or both and whether or not it's safe to give that along with carvedilol (Coreg), hydrochlorothiazide (HCTZ), furosemide (Lasix), losartan (Cozaar), and diltiazem (Cardizem). Know how your blood pressure pills work. Maybe I'm a little into this because I work on a cardiac floor, but I can tell you that a lot of patients get really sick because some nurse doesn't understand the differences between them and proceeds to give eight different antihypertensives at one time. A lot of patients don't understand their blood pressure pills. Antihypertensives and antiarrhythmics cause a lot of problems, so learn about them and respect them. Pharm is a lot of rote memorization, but understanding A & P will make it easier to learn (i.e., alpha blockers vs. beta blockers and how these affect patients with asthma).

Gerontology (Gero). The study of old people. It's a good idea to pay attention in this class because unless you go straight into pediatrics, the majority of people you'll take care of will be old. At the time I took this course, my grandfather was 96. I helped look after him a little bit in his final days, so this course really struck a chord with me. It's essential to not throw old people to the curb just because they're old. They've paved the way and are valuable members of society. I think their latter years should be as sweet as the former. The 70 or 80-year-old body works much differently from the 20 or 30- something-year-old's body. Currently on my nursing floor, I'd say the average age of my patients is 70. They are a challenging group to care for, but funny too and very sweet. Learn about their needs and how to meet them. And always remember that you might be in their shoes one day too. My parents are in their 60s now and every time I take care of an older person, I can't help but think of them. You're going to be caring for someone's mother or father, grandmother or grandfather. Care and be respectful. Patience is a necessity with this group too.

In Gero, we had to write a paper for which we had to interview two elderly people (over age 65), and write about two important issues they face and how they handle them. I interviewed a lady and a gentleman on two different ends of my street. It was very interesting to hear them discuss how they spend their time, how they planned for retirement, and the unique problems they face because of age. I would have included the paper for you, but unfortunately, I'm not able to hunt it down.

Adult Health Nursing-Body Defense Mechanisms. This was the course where we studied what they call "Med Surge (Medical-Surgical)" or I guess you could say basic nursing. We studied how to take care of the patient with cancer, the patient with orthopedic injuries, and the patients with diabetes. For the clinical portion of this course I was on an orthopedic floor, where patients went to recover from hip replacements, knee replacements, spinal fusions, and other musculoskeletal surgeries. I've always been fascinated by bones and ligaments. Pain management was important in this setting, as you can imagine.

I remember caring for a gentleman who had hyperextended his neck, which led to a cervical spine (neck) fracture. He had to get surgery to repair the bones in his neck. It's a miracle the man wasn't paralyzed. He got his injury at a party trying to do some sort of flip while intoxicated. He was an interesting character. I remember the thrill of taking out his Foley catheter (the first one I'd ever removed) and felt especially proud when he said he didn't feel a thing. It was also very rewarding to help him walk for the first time after his surgery.

Getting these orthopedic/post-operative patients moving as soon as possible is extremely important during the recovery process. It's fun to help relieve people's pain too. My advice to students in this type of rotation is to try to spend a little extra time understanding the pain meds you encounter. Roxicodone, morphine, Dilaudid, tramadol, and Percocet are neat drugs. It's also pretty cool to see how they affect people differently. For the clinical rotation of this course I remember doing a presentation about infection control in the hospital. It was an easy project, like most are in nursing school, but just a little time consuming. We also had to write a paper about a certain population or culture of patients. See appendix.

Psychiatric/Mental Health Nursing. As you can imagine, this is an interesting one. Psych (short for "psychiatric") nursing deals with helping people who have any and all types of mental illness. I'll say up front here it's not a field I've ever been interested in working in. Once you go through your clinical in psych, maybe you'll see why. Psych nurses spend a lot of time doing what I considered babysitting. To me, it looked like they just passed meds, told patients to go to their therapy sessions, and then charted the rest of the shift on what the patients were doing. B-O-R-I-N-G.

To prep for this clinical at a psychiatric facility, we had to learn how to do a mental health assessment, which meant asking all sorts of questions to see if our patient was suicidal, homicidal, depressed, or just potentially psychotic. We did this in clinical, each on a different patient. And yep, you guessed it, we had to turn it into a paper. I interviewed a 50-some year-old lady who was depressed and had overdosed on alcohol.

Psych nursing was simply just sad to me. One of the saddest things about this place was that it had a children's unit.

Apparently, there are some kids out there whose parents can't handle the temper tantrums and screaming and all. And then there was an adolescent unit where some delinquent kids settled. It was really sad talking to the young people. I could see how much damage is done when kids come from jacked-up homes—kids get abused sexually or they witness the abuse of a parent. Just one time messes a kid up for life. It's a hard thing to fix. Broken families often yield wounded people, which often contributes to a shattered society.

In this rotation, I even met a mom who tried to kill herself. She had a husband who loved her and two young kids. I remember asking her how that would affect her family. It seems a lot of people with psych issues can only see themselves and their own problems. I can't say for sure because I've never been there. But, I am pretty sure that most people have at least someone (even if it's a dog) in their life that cares deeply and would be very sad if they were gone.

The psych nursing textbook is one I do recommend reading. Mental illness is so interesting. I realized when getting into all of the different disorders that half the people I know, including myself, have at least some attributes found in personality disorders. In psych, you'll learn about bipolar, schizophrenia, anxiety disorders, phobias, and narcissistic personalities. And then you start to understand (briefly) the minds of criminals. It's quite fascinating.

One of the main reasons I really didn't care for psych nursing is that it seemed like all the nurses would do to help people was give them meds and those patients really couldn't function without them. The major problem to me was that they didn't seem to function *on* them either. So many of the patients in that psych facility walked around so doped up on psychiatric medications. Note: Read about and learn your psych meds too. They're very interesting and so are their side effects. Learn about lithium, Xanax, Wellbutrin, Cogentin, Paxil, and Prozac. You will see them in the real world.

Even if you don't go into psych, you'll deal with a lot of mentally ill and just flat out "strange" people. It's sad but true. And it's also interesting to look at how these people often fall into the gaps. What is society supposed to do with mentally ill people who can't afford the help of a psychiatrist or get turned away from mental health facilities that are too full as it is? Do we throw them back on the street and just hope they don't hurt other people? Do we put them in jail? It's certainly something to think about.

I often think about the young man in December 2012 who walked into a school in Newtown, Connecticut and murdered 20 innocent little kids and six adults just days before Christmas. He shouldn't have been able to do that. Was he insane, demon-possessed, or both? And I think about Columbine, the Navy Yard, Virginia Tech, and the Colorado movie theatre shootings, as well as all the others. Mental illness affects a lot of people. Mentally unstable individuals shouldn't be able to hurt innocent people trying to go about their lives. But is there a way to help them live productive and meaningful lives? Can we prevent mental illness in the first place?

It is easy to see how mental health nurses can play a role in public policy. Lawmakers need to be in touch with nurses and others who work first-hand with the mentally ill. Mental health is just as important as physical health. People are made up of mind, body, and spirit. If one's ill, the other two won't work. The three must exist in harmony and work together. What good is it to have a healthy body but a rotten mind? One of the reasons I love nursing is that it forces you to examine these difficult issues. It's about people. I applaud those who do or eventually will work in mental health nursing.

I also want to comment that psych nursing teaches you some really useful things you can learn in whatever field of nursing you go into. Pay special attention to the chapter/topic of safety when working with this population. As nurses, we're always taught that the patient's safety is our top priority. But, if you're anything like me, you also care about your own safety. One of the best tips I got was to always put yourself between the patient and the door. The patient should never be between you and the door. Mentally ill people can be violent. And strong. Not a good combination if you're 5'2 110-pounds and you just happen to be assigned to a psych patient during a manic episode. My point: Watch out for yourself.

Nursing Research. This one is similar to the agony of writing care plans, especially if you get stuck with that teacher who sounds bored with the subject matter herself. This is the class where you, as stated, learn about nursing research. I must admit that it is actually somewhat (very) useful if you really think about it. There are such things as nurse researchers. Any type of nurse can be involved in research—floor nurses, nurse managers, and nurse practitioners (NPs). They find issues in the real world of nursing and conduct studies to figure out what works best in the real world. You'll often hear the term "evidence-based practice." The way things are done in hospitals are usually done that way because some team somewhere tried to figure out the best way of doing it. By "best," I mean most efficient, safest, most cost-effective, most productive, etc. It's pretty cool if you think about it. Once you take this class, you realize why they made you take statistics as a prerequisite to your program. Once you start reading nursing research articles and you start learning all the terms (sample size, N, limitations, etc.), that little bell will ring in your mind. I'm also very grateful for people who do nursing research. To me, it sounds like a big headache because to do research right, you have to understand statistics as well as the proper way of actually doing a study. There are a lot of things that can interfere with your results when you're a researcher and you have to be aware of them.

We did spend a lot of time up front in this class learning the terms, so yeah, it's a good idea to read your textbook. But, I will say that if you're pressed for time, this is a class in which you can afford to just "skim" the book. Mainly, know the highlighted/bolded terms. They'll help you. We also learned a lot about American Psychological Association or APA format in this class. My teacher was a stickler for it. Learn APA format or whatever standard your program uses for citing your sources when you write papers. It is used in graduate school too, so it won't go away.

I wasn't a fan of how this class was set up in my program. Our grade was largely determined by papers we wrote—as a group. Group work. Blah. It is extremely difficult to assemble eight to ten different people who work, have families, and all live 45 minutes apart from each other at the same time several times a week in order to work on a paper. It's ridiculous. We wrote multiple lengthy papers in this class as a group. Groups were assigned at the start of the semester and we did not get to pick our members. One of the papers written for this course required us to analyze research studies pertinent to a particular topic of research in nursing. Our group chose pressure ulcers. We each had to find a research article and critique it. We had to evaluate how well the authors stated the purpose of the research, whether or not the sample size was clearly defined, and whether the research actually answered the question at hand. I'm getting bored just thinking back on this class. It was a lot of work. It's hard to write a paper with 10 different people. Hopefully one person in the group is a good leader and will step up and take the reins. Hopefully there's a grammar/APA nut, a person who likes to find articles, and a person who likes to organize the flow of the paper. If each person has a job, it makes things a little bit smoother.

Overall, I will say that Nursing Research is a beneficial course. It's one of those things that sets BSN students apart from the basic RN or LPN students. Think of this class as just another required item on your checklist to becoming a nurse. It can be dry at times, but do learn what makes a research article good or bad and whether or not you would use it to support your point in a paper. Also, if you go into hospital management or administration one day, differentiating between good research and bad research can help you decide what policies should be implemented in your workplace and which ones shouldn't be. Additionally, if you look at the grand scheme of things, it could save lives, improve patient and staff experiences at your hospital, and ultimately put more cash in your pocket. See where I'm headed?

Therapeutic Diets II. This class is very similar to Therapeutic Diets I. Again, it's easy. I think in this semester, we studied more of the diets that help people with the particular diseases we covered in Nursing 340/341. Basically, you can memorize this in one day and come out okay. Don't kill yourself in this class; in the real world, you'll have dieticians and nutritionists and diabetes educators who get paid to write menus up for your patients and to educate them on what they should and shouldn't eat. But nonetheless, it's helpful information for you as the RN as well.

Care of the Childbearing Family/Clinical Management of the Childbearing Family. Obstetrics (or OB, women's health and reproduction) isn't my specialty right now in life; it's not even that area of nursing that I was super attracted to while in school. I must say, though, that this is a fascinating course. Conception and the whole human reproduction model is amazing. I really enjoyed reading the textbook in this class. This *is* a class for which you should read. There's a lot of numbers and times and different things to memorize, like how long each stage of labor is and what the fetus' heart rate should be during each trimester, and how the female body changes throughout pregnancy.

I took the clinical portion of this course at a major hospital in my city. We spent one week in the Labor and Delivery area, some time in the newborn nursery, and some time on the mother/baby unit. I must say that Labor and Delivery is pretty sweet. I understand that many people are horrified and completely grossed out by watching childbirth. To me though, it is one of the most magnificent things on the earth to witness. New life.

The first labor and delivery that I saw was that of a young 18-year-old. I remember talking to the girl in between her contractions. Being the naïve nursing student I was at the time, I didn't even realize that she was in labor. She took it like a champ. She was a high school student and told me she'd have to go to school at night in order to finish. The girl had no pain meds during labor. She seemed to only push a couple times, she screamed and huffed and puffed, had her legs open. The female doctor came in and I remember her saying, "Let's have a baby." Bam, the 18-year-old girl gave birth to a baby girl. A classmate and I stood in the corner and cried. It was amazing. The girl's mother and grandparents were there. I remember talking to the girl right after she delivered and asked if I could get her anything. She said she was starving and wanted a burger. I learned that they don't let women in labor eat just in case they have to end up getting a C-section (it's a risk with anesthesia). So, I went downstairs and got her a burger, fries, and a lemonade. That made her happy and I felt good being able to help her.

During that rotation, I tried to take time to read charts. I still to this day could sit at the computer forever (because it's so nice to sit) and read up on patients. I always try to find out where they come from, where they live, and what their home life and work life are like. It shapes them. I remember one day in L & D, I looked at records of the women expected to give birth. I was heartbroken to see the reality that only two out of the 10 were married. I've always believed that sex is very sacred and that it is to be between a man and a woman who are married to each other. To make life with someone is not something to be taken lightly.

The labor and delivery portion was my favorite part of this rotation. I got to see a C-section, which was pretty awesome too. That girl was young as well. She got an epidural before the procedure started. She had to lean over and the anesthesiologist inserted this long needle into her back. She laid down on the table and the doc cut her stomach open, reached in, and pulled a little baby boy out. They sat him on another table and then the neonatologists came in and examined him. That girl's C-section was scheduled. I discovered a little bit about that mom by reading her chart and talking to her. Apparently her home was a correctional center and this was her fifth child. There was a man present when she had the C-section; I assumed it was the baby's father. To me, it seemed like the girl was so nonchalant about everything.

If nothing else, the maternity rotation will open your eyes to some deeper issues faced in our society. I said in the Psych section that nursing makes you think. Here again, nursing makes you think. I remember watching all these babies be born to young mothers. In many cases, the baby's father was not there. A lot of the moms I witnessed give birth were still in high school. They had no source of income, no education. One would have to ask where the money comes from to take care of that new baby. Who pays the doctor who delivered the baby? What kind of environment is that child going to grow up in—with no father; a young, poor, uneducated, unemployed mother? And what about the mother? Will she be able to finish high school and raise a baby by herself? Should she receive a monthly check from taxpayers to pay her rent and buy groceries for her child? And what about the absent father? Should he be held liable for not contributing to the well-being of his offspring? What if he is also young, poor, uneducated, and unemployed? What if this couple has another child at the same hospital? Who pays the bill to the hospital staff (including the nurses involved in the delivery)? What if the girl here is being sexually assaulted and has no way out? I don't mean to step on any toes here at all; I just want to give you a taste of the things that nursing makes you think about.

To end this section on a lighter note, I want to share a funny story. One day, I was making my rounds on my assigned patients on the Mother & Baby unit. I peeked into one room and saw a young woman standing there. Her belly was distended, so I asked,

"Oh, when's your baby due?" She told me that she had already had her baby. Doh. I was not aware that post-partum women tend to hold on to a little bit of weight in the midsection after the delivery. I felt a little embarrassed, but again, as I said before, L&D/Mother-Baby is not my area of expertise.

Adult Health Nursing II Organ/System + Clinical. Adult Health II was where we learned about hypo/hyperthyroidism, congestive heart failure, pancreatitis, COPD, diabetes, and pretty much all of the ins and outs of those conditions, because it is a lot of what you'll see in nursing. I think I got a B in this course. I remember our tests were just 50 questions, multiple choice. It was tough to get an A. We used the same textbook for this portion of Med-Surge as we had used in Adult Health I. Read the textbook. Looking back now, all of what we learned in this course makes so much more sense now that I've actually seen it and I deal with it every day. The teacher for my course worked as an RN at some hospital in the area, so she was knowledgeable, but she liked to read from the powerpoint. Again, you have to teach yourself, or get in a good study group if that's your thing. Understand your meds and how they work. Try to refresh your memory on A & P stuff because it will make these conditions a lot more understandable and you won't be trying to memorize every little thing.

The clinical portion of this course was the part of nursing school where I cried. You'll always hear people moan about how hard nursing school is, and I didn't really think it was, until I got to this course. I am pretty sure it was because of my instructor (of course it couldn't have been my own fault). Anyhow, I think it was an eight or ten-week rotation. I was on a cardiac/telemetry unit. I think about eight or nine other students were in my clinical group. This clinical started out okay because I was lucky enough to have my "observation" time during the first two weeks. This means I was sent to the cath lab (where they put stents in people's hearts to open them up after a heart attack) or to the endoscopy lab to watch stress tests or colonoscopies, respectively. So, for the first two weeks, I didn't even really have to do the pre-clinical paperwork. It was nice.

We had to do our usual pre-clinical paperwork the day before our actual clinical day, which was once a week. This pre-clinical day was Monday for me. I'd drive from home, leaving the house around 7:15 am and drive to class, sit in lecture for about two hours, drive to the gym, then drive another 40 minutes to the hospital to get my patient assignment and start working on my pre-clinical paperwork. My instructor didn't post patient assignments until 2 P.M. sometimes. I would get out there and get to work as soon as possible. She'd text us the room number of our patient and we'd have to go in and log in to the computer and learn basically every single thing there was to know about that patient. At the start of this rotation, I was laid-back. Besides, in my mind, I shouldn't have to spend three hours looking up stuff about my patient before actually meeting him or her. Again, that's not how it works in the real world. It's so interesting to write this retrospectively because all the stuff that seemed so hard and mind-boggling back then is quite simple now because I do it every day or work with someone who knows what I don't. We had to fill out this long form of things about the patient, including why he or she was admitted, labs, why some lab values were off, the patient's history, etc. Oh, and meds. We had to write down/type every single medication the patient was on, why he/she got it, its mechanism of action, drug interactions, side effects, and side effects. It was basically like copying the drug handbook. We had to type all this stuff up and e-mail it to the instructor by midnight. And then in the morning we'd get drilled.

Once my two-week observation time was over and I got on the floor for clinical, it seems like my instructor was intent upon making me suffer. I remember her "cracking down" and saying how lousy of a job all of us were doing and how if we continued on in our sub-par performance, we would not be prepared for Critical Care. I thought I was a perfectionist, but soon learned I wasn't. I found out my peers were working on their pre-clinical reports for about eight hours, while I was working on them three hours max. They would type up these unbelievable reports—the "pre-clinical paperwork". Uhhh. Some of my peers would have just pages and pages and pages of information about their patient. There was a section on pathophysiology, where we had to give a "brief" summary of the patient's major condition. For labs, we'd have to say why we thought the patient's lab value was abnormal, if it was abnormal. We'd have to write down every thing about every medication—why it was prescribed, how it was given, how often it was given, side effects, drug interactions, etc. It was nuts. I remember even saying that I stop my work at three hours because sleep was important to me. My instructor somehow vividly remembered me saying that and seemed to use it against me. I still did my work thoroughly, but I just thought I was a student for a reason and that getting a good night's rest before a clinical day would do me more good than staying up all night in order to rewrite the pathophysiology or medication textbooks.

I remember my clinical instructor saying how she let me do the observation portion early in the rotation because she wasn't concerned about me having a hard time with the clinical aspects since I worked at a nursing home at the time and was supposedly familiar with the medical environment and working with patients. Apparently she had overestimated me. I had never given meds through a PEG tube (a tube surgically placed through the abdomen into the stomach for the purpose of feeding people who cannot swallow) or administered antibiotics intravenously or even mixed antibiotics or given a subcutaneous injection or drawn up insulin. She grilled me on each of these things.

I remember early in the clinical she assigned a very challenging (high acuity) patient to me. He had a lot of stuff going on with him, sort of the typical patient I'm used to working with now. He had a ton of medications that needed to be given, couldn't talk, was confused, and was on isolation for C-diff (a form of diarrhea). He had a PEG tube as well as a Foley catheter (a tube that goes into the urethra to drain the bladder). I remember my instructor took the lead in crushing his pills and doing all the work for me. She moved around his room frantically and appeared more stressed out than any of the students. We were also behind schedule that day. It was a really bad day. I remember leaving that clinical day thinking about how my grade in the class was probably not in the best standing and also about how much I needed to learn.

At the halfway point in this clinical, we had to meet with the instructor individually to be evaluated. Me and a couple others were singled out and we had to go to her office. I had gotten a text message from her one afternoon saying that I needed to see her in her office the next day. I knew what it was for. When I met with her, she told me that I was being put on "clinical caution." Basically, I wasn't living up to the expectations that had been set for a junior nursing student and I was at risk of failing. Sometimes I wondered if clinical instructors were required by their superiors to put a certain number of students on clinical caution in order to meet some quota, to make the nursing program appear hard. The other kid who was put on clinical caution had once been a corpsman in the military. His wife was pregnant and he had a lot of stuff going on in his life. He seemed competent to me.

Anyhow, after this little setback, I got to enjoy a week of spring break. I told myself that I would whip it into high-gear for the next four weeks or so and do what I had to do in order to pass. I spent some extra time in the skills lab at school, watched a bunch of YouTube videos on how to give injections, and finally watched the skills videos that came with some textbooks. And yes, I did start spending even more time on the pre-clinical work. I remember one night, I stayed up pretty late typing and researching. When I finally went to lay down, I couldn't even sleep because I had so much anxiety about whether or not I'd do well. I got up and watched some more videos on how to do sub-q injections. I used an ink pen as a pretend needle.

That next day, I left the house extremely early to drive to the hospital for clinical. I think it was something like 5:30 am when I *got* there. I got there super early because I couldn't sleep and I wanted to see the latest in the chart on the patient. I also wanted to talk to some nurses and ask questions that I didn't want to ask my instructor. I remember my instructor asking me first thing in the morning something about a fistula and she asked me if I had looked it up. And of course, that was the one thing that I had *not* looked up. It was a blow because I felt like I had worked so hard all night and I got slammed first thing in the morning. Anyhow, as those few weeks went on, I did improve. My instructor had enough of a heart to say so. I remember the first time she saw me draw up heparin or insulin and I had no idea what size needle to use or even how to draw the thing up. Going to the skills lab had helped too. I also had a classmate who was kind enough to help me sort of cram right before I had to demonstrate how to mix an IV med in its pouch and how to connect the tubing. I thanked her later for helping me survive that test. When the Adult Health II clinical finally came to an end, I was so glad. I even passed, with a B. The two others who had been put on clinical caution passed too, but it did make one friend of mine consider quitting the program. I tried to talk her out of it but to no avail.

See the Appendix for a sample of pre-clinical work.

Pharmacology II. As you can imagine, pharmacology is a broad field. It takes two semesters to pretty much just pop the top off of all you need to know. Pharm II was no harder than Pharm I and looking back now, I don't remember what was covered in each half. I think our instructor (the same one for both portions) just split the book in half for each semester. There were some meds that we hardly discussed and then there were some sections about which she said, "Make sure you guys read the section on such and such because it will be on the test." Pharm is really really cool and it is important to know the basics of how medicines work. Again, use flash cards. A lot of this course is memorization. But at the same time, try not to memorize everything. A cool trick is to think about suffixes on meds, like "-olol" and "-thiazide" and "-cin." This will help you to learn categories of drugs like beta blockers, diuretics, and antibiotics. If you can learn the classes and just a little bit about how the meds in those classes work, you'll be okay. Don't be worried about learning everything because after you've worked a year on your first job in whatever specialty it is, things will make a LOT more sense. I can tell you more about Metoprolol, Zosyn, Protonix, and Dilaudid now than I ever could have when I was in school because I give them to patients several times a day every day. And at your job, you'll be able to look things up. We have something called "Micromedex" that shows up as a link in the Medication Administration Record (MAR) underneath each med. You can click on it and find whatever you need to know about each med. Anyhow, Pharm II was easy.

Therapeutic Diets III. Again, refer to the first two portions I wrote about earlier. Same teacher, skim the powerpoint notes, memorize. Easy. Pay special attention to diets for kidney and heart failure patients, because you actually will see that in the real world. Learn about diabetes too.

Nursing Care of Infants and Children/Clinical Management. This is the course we referred to as "Peds" (short for pediatrics). It's interesting stuff. I found this course to be a little more academically challenging, probably because I never officially held a babysitting job growing up and was never in a hurry to supervise children or to have my own. In this course, you learn about all the stages of young people. We started studying them from birth up to age 21 (young adult). The definition of "kid" or "child" seems to vary across the board. Anyhow, I highly recommend getting a pediatric pocket guide with all the stages of development and special numbers that you'll need to know. Carry it with you to clinical. In this class, it's a very good idea to read the book. There's a lot of information and lots of reading. You learn about how kids see the world, how they learn and interpret things in different stages, as well as medical conditions that are unique to them, like ear infections, intussusception, and genetic problems. You also learn about safety for kids, which is important.

Mothers have an advantage in this class. I've always had a hard time learning what's normal for kids. I've also found it hard, and still do, to look at a kid and try to guess how old he or she is. But kids are fascinating. This class offers a lot of neat information. Yes, I memorized a lot of things, especially numbers. We also had to memorize at what age infants should be rolling onto their stomach, holding things, and walking. Pediatrics is not my forte, so this was hard for me to get into. One of my friends had had a baby right around the time I was in the childbearing course of the nursing program, so I would think of him as well as all the other kids in church that I did know and try to think of what they were doing in order to help me in this class. If you have a child of your own or a niece or nephew or a kid you watch that is developing "normally," use him or her as your model to help you in this class.

Again, our tests in here were 50 questions, maybe a little more at times, mostly multiple choice. My instructor in this course was pretty good, and her lectures were more than just reading off the powerpoint. But still, read the book before lecture and then come with questions. Depending on what type of learner you are, I recommend typing notes during lecture. It's quicker than hand writing and you have to think about something and slightly process it as you put it down on paper, so it helps reinforce the material. Unless you go work in peds right out of school, you're going to forget a lot of stuff you learn in this class. Don't worry a ton about seeing lots of peds questions on the NCLEX; at least I didn't see many.

Luckily, there is a children's hospital close by. It's basically where all the kids go, or at least should go, to get care. From my experience, if you send your newborn to the ER at any other hospital for care, they're going to tell you to go to the children's hospital to get the best care. The people at children's hospitals specialize in kids; the other hospitals don't. I saw some neat stuff in this rotation. We floated to a different area each week. One week, I took care of a girl who was about 10-years-old. She had a sad story. She had cerebral palsy and had come from a nursing facility because of respiratory failure. She needed total care. I remember doing incontinence care (cleaning up urine and stool) for her. I still sometimes think about her and her future. I wonder about her parents, who I never met.

Another week, I cared for a 6-year-old girl who had a staph infection on her skin—all over her body. It was from eczema. The poor girl itched all over. She was an interesting case. I actually used her for my case study that we had to do at the end of the rotation. I remember one doctor telling that girl's mother that she might have to go to some special camp-type place in another state in order to get treatment for her skin condition because it was so severe. I remember interacting with this girl and thinking about how different kids are from adults when it comes to being a patient. They're shy and it seems to me they wouldn't be quite as demanding as adults. This kiddo played with her doll while doctors came in to see her.

Another week I worked with the babies. I took care of one who was a few weeks old. His mom was 16. The baby (the newborn) was being treated for meningitis. I remember only changing his diaper, as the peds rotation involved mostly observation. With this kid, I spent most of the time talking to his young mom trying to convince her to stay in school and such. I gave her some information about nursing school because she said she wanted to be a nurse. I told her about the local career training center and classes offered by the community college. It's always saddened me to see young teen moms as I discussed previously. I do wonder how that young girl is doing now and whether or not her child even gets to see his father.

 I also later heard that the nurse was going in to the baby's room and walked in on the 16-year-old mom and her boyfriend having relations. Welcome to nursing.

 There was another young kid I felt really sorry for. Apparently he had just been diagnosed with type I diabetes. Know your pathophys; type I is very different from type II diabetes. He was a young kid and had been out playing soccer. His mom was there with him and I remember they were talking about his dad. It seemed that his parents were really supportive. The family had something huge on their plates with the diagnosis. It was sad. I really wanted to help them.

Just on the other side of the curtain, another kid I observed had a huge head. His condition was called hydrocephalus. He had a shunt in his head that was used to move excess fluid. His parents stayed by his side. I can't imagine the feeling of having a sick child.

There were these two other kids, a brother and his older sister. They were laying in the bed together; she was there to comfort him. I had to give him a flu shot, which was the first intramuscular injection I'd ever given. The poor kid. His big sister held his hand. He closed his eyes and screamed as I stuck the sterile needle into his little deltoid. It was quick and done. We all praised him afterward for doing so well. Intramuscular injections still freak me out. Sometimes it seems I can feel the thick needle hit the patient's bone and then it has to be pulled back slightly. It usually stings too. Creepy.

For one week of this clinical, the nursing program sent us to a day care in a neighboring city. We had to go there and observe kids, the 3-year-olds to be exact. They were an intriguing bunch to say the least. I remember one Caucasian little boy with dark hair. He was content to just sit on the carpet with a finger up his nose. I was really amused when he then proceeded to examine the retrieved contents from his nostrils and then place that finger in his mouth. Apart from observing nose-picking rituals, I had snack time with the kids, played at recess with them, and read with them. They were so welcoming and trusting. They were in their own world. Fun was what mattered to them. God bless day care workers, though. I couldn't do it.

Adult Nursing III/Clinical Management of Adults III.
This is a really fun course because it is the course in critical care. A lot of people, or at least I, get a little tingly feeling inside when thinking about "critical care." If you tell people, "I'm an ICU nurse" or "I work in the ER (Emergency Room)," many assume you're an adrenaline or trauma junkie. They also lend you respect because of your title; at least that's been my observation.

This was a very enjoyable, yet time-consuming and demanding class. My instructor, whom I really respect, is a wife, mother of two, and practicing ER nurse. She called herself a trauma junkie. As a matter of fact, I remember sitting in nursing school orientation the week before classes started and hearing her introduce herself. She was very energetic all the time, like she'd had too much coffee or something. Or maybe she was just passionate about her job. I think it was both, but more of the latter. She got up and said, "The more blood and guts, the more I wanna be there!" She was a phenomenal lecturer. Her class was not one I could easily fall asleep in. To encourage us to read our textbook each week, she might or might not have a quiz before class on the reading material, so we had better come prepared. If we did well enough on the quizzes, they could help out with the overall grade in the class. I think we had a total of 10 throughout the 16-week semester, and she dropped the two lowest grades. It's very important to read in this class. And read slowly. As I said earlier, you'll be grateful that you paid attention in your A & P course because it will make critical care a lot easier if you're familiar with your basic anatomy and how the organ systems work. This class is hard. Dr. Linn was tough. She wanted us to know what we were doing. She wanted us to be competent. I sort-of felt sorry for the kids that had her for clinical, but now looking back, I think she was kind-hard on them just for the sake of making them better. (She wasn't mean like my clinical instructor in Adult Health II).

We covered so many cool topics in her class. We covered a

lot, so she talked fast. This was the class where I really just brought my laptop and typed while I listened to her. She was so intriguing that she was easy to follow. She had one of those voices that stood out, like Woody (Tom Hanks) on Toy Story. I could hear her voice while taking a test. She recorded her lectures on "Classroom Capture" and then uploaded them onto the course website. If I remember right, she did something tricky, though, to where if a student skipped class, she couldn't listen to the lecture online. I never really considered myself much of an auditory learner, but for her class, in the middle to later portion of the semester, after struggling to get above an 85 on her exams, I took the advice of classmates who were doing well, and I started listening to her lectures. Listening and looking at the notes simultaneously helped to get things in my head. My exam grades improved by about a whopping two points, I suppose a reflection of the fact that I'm not much of an auditory learner. I don't think I spent tons of time rereading chapters because her lectures were very thorough, I took good notes, and she covered the meat of what would be on the exams.

What made exams hard in this class was the types of

questions. A lot of the questions tested the students' ability to prioritize. To know if the patient with issue A should be helped before the patient with issue B should be helped, it was imperative to understand each condition and the complications associated with each one. The questions made us think. For nearly every question, we had to ask ourselves a couple of things. First, what's the definition of that condition? Second, will the patient die if I don't do something? What needs to be done? What needs to be done *first*? Dr. Linn taught us how to understand these things. Always think of airway first. Then circulation. Yes, we had to understand the basics and then be able to put it all together to answer each question correctly. It was what we called "higher level test questions."

In critical care, we covered all the intense, cool topics: shock; overdose; hypo/hyperthermia; stroke; burns; spinal cord injuries; organ transplantation; heart attack; aneurysms; trauma—motor vehicle accidents and the associated raccoon eyes, impalement, falls. During one lecture on trauma, Dr. Linn showed us some pictures of crazy real-life trauma patients, and she explained the stories behind them— an intoxicated boat-goer who had been impaled by a dock piling; a motorcycle crash victim; a bar-fight participant. Gruesome stuff. What amazes me even more is that there's real trauma doctors who get called to a room and they see some of that stuff. They have to figure out how to fix it. It's amazing.

Another lecture we had was from a lady who was head of the burn center in Washington, D.C. She shared some pictures too. Unbelievable stuff. She told us to not become burn nurses if we didn't like seeing people hurt. There were pictures of lineman, the guys that work on power lines, that had been electrocuted. There were pictures of baby's legs that had been placed in scolding hot water by their own abusive parents. There were firefighters that had been burned. There were chemical burns. Some burns had to be fixed by plastic surgeons. We learned about different treatments for the different types of burns. There's also a huge emotional healing part involved with burn patients because physical appearance is often distorted. My favorite thing was seeing before and after pictures of burn patients who had been through a recovery program. They had their lives restored. Beautiful.

Another lecturer we had was a guy from the organ

transplantation organization. We discussed the definition of "brain dead" and different neurological scores associated with that as well as hospital policies, ethics, and family issues associated with the topic of brain death. There's a lot of fascinating research out there about brain death too. Organ donation can really help people. If you go on to work in a hospital, you will work with organ donation organizations. People die. It's part of nursing.

Even if you don't end up in a trauma setting (you at least are not likely to start there), the information you go over in this class is helpful for daily life. You never know where you'll be when someone complains of chest pain or experiences stroke symptoms, needs CPR, or has frostbite. You'll learn some little helpful tips you can take with you.

I spent the clinical portion of this course at an independent hospital in my area. Again, another hike in terms of driving. It took me about 40 minutes to get out there. This rotation went quickly; it was just six weeks and we went twice a week. I spent the first bit in the ICU. One week, I had a lady with pancreatitis. I actually had her twice throughout the rotation. Other patients were septic and needed special drugs called vasopressors to keep their blood pressure up. I think another lady had had abdominal surgery for something and had been intubated for some reason. She was on propofol, what I always think of as "the Michael Jackson drug." Other patients were there because they had survived a stroke but were in bad shape. One lady had been in that ICU for months. She was unresponsive and had the fixed pupils. There were obvious end-of-life issues that needed to be addressed with her, but no family could be found. She was still legally married but it seemed that her estranged husband could not be found. I don't know what ever happened to her.

As I said earlier, I thought the ICU was kind-of slow. One day all we did really was adjust IV pumps according to patient's blood pressures. We got to sit a lot. I think a lot of ICU work is in the head. ICU nurses have to think and use a lot of nursing judgment because doctors leave pretty wide parameters in their orders. They must decide what's best for the patient. That's why a lot of new nurses don't start in the ICU. You need to know what you're doing. Also, respiratory equipment can be intimidating. Even though you have respiratory therapy staff, you're on standby when they're not around.

The ICU was so different to me because patients didn't talk and interact like I was used to. Assessments are a lot different. As you can imagine, ICU patients are usually in bad shape—if there's a place for a tube, there usually is a tube (Foley catheters in the urethra, nasogastric tubes in the nose, percutaneous endoscopic gastrostomy (PEG) tubes in the stomach, rectal tubes in the rectum of course, tracheostomies (traches) in the throat). The really sick patients are on some pretty hefty drugs, like propofol, so that they won't pull those tubes out—especially if they're on a ventilator. So instead of having a patient interact with you, the conversation is interpretive. If your patient can't talk to you, you can still talk to them. You as the nurse are responsible for reading what the patient is communicating to you via vital signs, responses to drugs, and pupils. You assess their pupils to see if the patient is neurologically intact. When you shine a light at the pupils and they don't change, that's bad. It's also bad if you see the eyes move in opposite directions.

In the critical care course, we had to present a topic at the end of the semester to our peers. My group spoke on heart attack—basic info. We also had to write a case study, in which we picked a very sick patient and wrote all about him/her. I've included this paper for you (see Appendix). For the lecture portion of the course, we had to write about organ transplantation (also included in the Appendix). This was probably the most challenging paper I wrote in nursing school simply because Dr. Linn was the grader. By the way, I think I got an 87 or an 89 on it, which my peers said was decent for a Dr. Linn grade. I of course, would have liked an A, but then again, I was no longer a perfectionist.

Community Health Nursing I. This was another one of those classes where we had to do some group work. The bulk of the grade in the class was based off a group presentation (and paper) done at the end of the semester. We had some lectures we had to go to as well, but I don't think we had any tests in here. One thing that was nice about this course was that we actually got to *do something* as opposed to just sitting and listening to a bunch of theory (which we still did some). In the classroom, we learned about HealthyPeople 2020, which is a government initiative to help people live healthier lives. We talked about different people groups and how they view health. Basically, this course was about us, on a small scale, going into the community and trying to teach and help people improve their health.

The instructor broke us all up into groups of about 10 and we were all assigned to different "demographic" groups spread throughout the city, such as single moms, the elderly, the and the obese. I was happy because I got to work with the group at a retirement/older people's living facility just a few blocks down from the school. The whole first semester of this course was about assessing our group (patient population), collecting and assessing data about them, and understanding their needs and desires for improving their own health. I believe we each had to log about 30 hours total throughout the semester of actually being on-site with this group. The first semester, our group spent a lot of time just talking with the residents and getting to know them. We did some creative things like make quizzes to see what they already knew about blood pressure, diabetes, nutrition, fitness, and the like. We assessed their blood pressures and heart rates. We figured out their ages and how long they normally exercised. It was clear to us early on that this group wanted to exercise more than they had been. At the end of the semester, we compiled all the data and simply wrote a paper about it, introduced our objective for the group, and then presented it in a big powerpoint presentation for the rest of our peers (and instructors) to see. It was rewarding getting to help people in the community.

Therapeutic Diets III. Again, refer to the first two sections on Therapeutic Diets. Same deal applies here.

The Final Semester of Nursing School

I made it. All of my time and hard work had led to the final semester. It started in early-mid January. Graduation was set for May 11th, and I was getting married at the end of May and then hopping on a boat to the Bahamas with my husband. The future was bright, yet there was still so much to be done. I remember Dr. Linn even warning us early on in the semester during the Transition course to not zone out because graduating did depend on successfully completing the requirements of that final semester. This semester was probably the most fun of all. The end was in sight. Also, I feel like the final semester of festivities, for the most part, actually mattered. It was like a giant springboard for becoming a "real" nurse.

Leadership, Management, & Professional Development. Yuck. This was another one of those courses that I feel we should have swapped with some hands-on time in the hospital. Yes, we got some good information in it, but again, it was sort of one of those things that is not really going to make sense or do much for you until you are a nurse manager. In this class, we met every other week for about three hours on a Monday afternoon. Our grade in the course consisted of three exams and I think a couple of random assignments. It was nothing too strenuous. The exam questions came right from the instructor's powerpoint notes. As a matter of fact, you can probably get by in here without reading the textbook. Oh, those random assignments were discussion board questions where we had to log in to the course website and respond to a question the teacher had posted about something we were supposed to read. So yes, it's probably not a bad idea to get the book. One option is to go half in with a friend and the two of you can share it.

In this class, we were introduced to several things regarding the workplace, like different models of nursing and staffing issues. We talked about different styles of leadership seen in nurse managers and different hospital/healthcare administrators, and how each one might run a nursing unit. We talked about how managers solve problems in the workplace—anything from conflict resolution to resource management and finances. These are problems that nurse managers (nurses with BSNs) deal with. In my opinion, I don't know why anyone would ever want to be a nurse manager. It's like being the president. I don't know how they sleep at night with all the responsibility they have. Uhhh.

Oh, the dreaded assignment in this class. It wasn't very difficult, just more annoying than anything. It was called the Root Cause Analysis. We had to read an article about an accident that occurred in a hospital which resulted in a baby's death. We had to trouble shoot the whole story and explore all the ways that the error could have been stopped. It's basically a quick little thing you can do in your head in about 10 minutes, but of course, they made us draw that out into a lengthy paper. In my opinion, this class should be put online.

*** Transition to Professional Nursing Practice. *** This is probably the best, most helpful and most worthwhile course in all of nursing school. Most of it is what's called the preceptorship. It's awesome. This class alternated with another course, so we only met every other week. Dr. Linn was in charge of this class, which is probably why it was so great. A huge chunk of our grade in here was the portfolio, which was both a paper and a website that each of us created to be like an online resume for ourselves. In the paper, we outlined how we met each competency of the program like professionalism, culture, and research. Spend time on this project—the website portion in particular, because I did use it for my job interview. It can help you stand out. Now whether my interviewers looked at it or not, I don't know. But it couldn't hurt.

In the classroom, we talked about the portfolio. Dr. Linn also helped us by giving us interviewing tips and the like. I really don't remember what else we did in the actual class other than that and talk about our portfolios. For this course, we were given a nursing instructor who was sort of like a mentor, or someone we could go to for help with questions. I was assigned to a very kind, laid-back woman.

The preceptorship is a fabulous way to network and get your foot in the door for a job right out of school. The previous semester in nursing school, Dr. Linn had each of us fill out a form where we could rank our preference as to what area of nursing we'd like to precept in (and perhaps work in right out of school). We could rank our top three. The areas listed included Intensive Care Unit (ICU), Emergency Department (ED), Medical Surgical (Med-Surge), Labor & Delivery (L & D), Cardiac/Telemetry, Stepdown, Mother/Baby, Oncology, Orthopedics, and Pediatrics (Peds). Again, you see that nursing is a great big world. We'd rank our preferences there, and then there was a spot on the form where we ranked the top three hospitals in the area where we'd like to precept. Then, I thought it was pretty cool that Dr. Linn even put on that form a spot for us to indicate what mattered more—being in a particular unit/specialty or being in a particular hospital. My first choice was the ED then Med-Surge and then Cardiac, if I remember correctly. Remember, I was still on my little buzz from getting to experience the ED during my critical care rotation. I said that location was more important to me than specialty/type of nursing. Again, I was tired of driving all over the place for rotations. Dr. Linn was awesome. She really fought to get each of us into the places we wanted to go. I remember that students had to have earned a good grade in critical care and received good evaluations from their clinical instructors in that course the previous semester if they wanted to precept in the ICU or ED because it was more competitive and a more serious / advanced place to start. Looking back now, I feel so fortunate because the preceptorship is how I landed my job—that I've been at for 13 months now (as of writing this). Dr. Linn explained to me that she had a hard time getting me into the ED at a nearby hospital. I was overall just happy that I only had to drive 10 minutes to get to the hospital I was eventually assigned to.

For the preceptorship, we got paired up with one nurse (maybe a max of two) that we had to shadow for a total of 120 hours over the course of six weeks. We could pretty much set that up however we wanted. A nurse at that hospital had to agree to precept us and we basically had to work off her schedule. We could bust those 120 hours out in three or four weeks if we wanted and we could do eight or 12-hour shifts, depending on what kind of schedule the preceptor worked. I think I got mine done in five weeks. I wasn't trying to kill myself. We also had to submit four clinical logs that documented what we had learned and how we had progressed as a student nurse through our experience.

The preceptorship was great. For me, it was mid-March through late April. I tried to get my hands on everything. I was fortunate enough to get a really great preceptor named Kelly. She had been a float pool nurse (meaning she worked all over the company's different facilities, wherever they needed her most; she was contracted to work at one hospital for a period of time, including the few weeks that I was with her for the preceptorship). I remember sitting outside the main nurses station on my first morning and hearing someone say, "There's Kelly." She was spirited first thing in the morning, had long brown hair and sparkly green eyes and carried only a plastic bag with her lunch in it. She smiled at me that first morning and truly welcomed me to tag along and learn. She even encouraged me to come in with a list of things I wanted to learn and see and do during that time so that she could make sure I had the opportunity to do so. [Side Note: Goals. Always set goals and know what you're trying to do or accomplish. It makes you so much more productive. That goes for anything—grocery shopping, working out, going to church, hanging out with a friend, whatever.] I had my list: I wanted to be in a code blue, learn how to start IVs and become comfortable at it, learn how to assess a patient properly, and get good at administering medications via multiple routes–pretty much learn all the stuff that I hadn't learned the past three years in the classroom.

Kelly reviewed my list and took me under her wing. She was so kind and warm and really liked to teach. She was excellent. The first week we started out, I just pretty much shadowed her and tagged along. We'd get to where each day I'd progress with the patient load (and that was what the school of nursing wanted us to do). By the end of the six-week period, we were supposed to be able to take on a full patient load and do what a real nurse does. I remember how nice it was having just one patient that I had to look after. Kelly had showed me the first week how to pull meds, how to assess, what to look for in the medical record, how to chart, and basically how to just work on the floor. I learned how some of the doctors work. I learned policies. I met other nurses. It was wonderful. We did EKGs, called doctors for orders and to notify them of lab values, dealt with difficult situations, and more.

My first day was hilarious. Looking back now, I see how much it truly reflects my home nursing floor. We went into a room to assess our patient who had been admitted for alcohol withdrawal. I can't remember his whole history, but he was indeed in withdrawal. He was a young skinny Caucasian guy, in his late 20s or early 30s. I looked around his room. He had an IV in his arm that was connected to a pump on a pole. He looked around the room, when suddenly, for some reason, probably because he wanted a drink, he took off full speed out of the room and ran down the hallway. Kelly chased him and tried to get him to stop running. I followed her. The patient approached the exit by the stairway, still attached to his IV pole, with his banana bag running (the banana bag is an IV bag that contains vitamins in it; alcoholics are typically malnourished because they just drink and they don't eat). He was at a dead end. We had all stopped at the small nurses station at the back of the floor. The guy looked around for a minute like a wild rabbit caught in a hunter's trap. Kelly was quick enough to get his IV fluid disconnected from him. Then he took off and bolted out the door and ran down the stairs. He was gone. Kelly, who was at that moment flustered and unfamiliar with the floor and the appropriate protocol, asked a nurse at the desk what to do. That nurse called a code purple—which means patient elopement. Security shows up to those. Within a few minutes, the patient was back up on the floor, accompanied by several officers. We gave him some Ativan and within a few minutes he was sound asleep in his room.

Another day there was an RRT, also known as a Rapid Response (Team). It was announced over the intercom. Everyone went rushing into the room at the end of the hallway to find a middle-aged obese female patient in the bed. She was winded and a little distraught, but she turned out okay. Apparently she had "vagaled down" (this refers to a maneuver in which someone bears down or holds their breath; it causes the heart rate to slow because of a complex interplay between the vagus nerve, acetylcholine, and the heart) while using the bedpan, causing her heart rhythm to flat line on the screen in the tele room. Harriett, the unit manager (and my future boss), was there in the room assisting, I guess partly because her office was right by that room. I was in the corner of the room. I heard Harriett say, "Rachel." I was reluctant to respond (she called me by the wrong name) to that although I had a feeling she was trying to get my attention. She wanted me to grab the bedpan from her. I stretched out a hand to take it. I only remember there being some dirty wet wipes in it, for which I was grateful. That rapid response ended on a positive note.

I thought it was cool that I got to be in there during that RRT. Kelly always tried to get me in a room whenever there was some action, especially during an RRT or a code blue. It's quite the experience and an excellent way to learn. That experience was awesome (although not incredibly eventful) because my face was seen by the manager of the floor. Cha-ching. One brownie point for me. ☺

One of the things I really liked about Kelly was that she wanted to get out of work on time. She would get after it all day long, organize her time, prioritize, jump in to assist me, and do whatever she had to do to be able to leave by 7:30 (or 3:30, if we were working an eight-hour shift). She showed me all kinds of shortcuts and tips to getting ahead and staying ahead. I'll go over all this later. At 7:00, we'd be at the front desk ready to give report for shift change.

Kelly was good at her job. She was kind and professional. It did however, comfort me to see her get frustrated and frazzled at times. It showed the reality of the job. Even the best nurses can feel stressed out or overwhelmed. I remember one day a cardiologist had made some smart comment along the lines of

"You don't know that and you're the patient's nurse?!" because he had asked a question that Kelly didn't know the answer to. Kelly was really offended by that because she knew (and I did too) that she was a good nurse. Doctors will sometimes ask you some really specific question about patient assessment or a med you gave 10 hours ago and if you can't remember or don't know off the top of your head, they seem to automatically conclude that you're incompetent. That cardiologist is still not one of my favorites to this day. Good thing I don't see him often.

I think one more thing that helped me with my preceptorship was that at the very end of it, I bought a thank you card from the hospital gift shop. I hand-wrote in it that I was grateful for the experience, that I really enjoyed the floor, and that I hoped to be a part of it in the near future. I put that card underneath Harriett's door on the last day of my preceptorship. And I bought Kelly a small gift to thank her. She had recommended me to the manager. Harriett had even mentioned to me one day that I should put in an application there since that floor was hiring. I made myself known to her. It helped me out just a few weeks later. I put my application in and had an interview with her and another manager there before

I even graduated.

Make the most of your preceptorship. Meet nurses who work that floor and ask them what they like and don't like about it. Ask them about their schedules, a normal day on the floor, and employee benefits. Observe the flow. See how things are done. Meet the secretary, doctors, respiratory therapists, housekeepers, and every other person you can meet. Get into every code blue and RRT that you can, even if you're just there in the corner to grab a bedpan like I was. Maybe you'll be lucky enough to do chest compressions. See all you can see, touch everything they'll let you touch, do whatever they'll let you do. Have fun. Learn everything you can. Make yourself known to the clinical coordinator and the nurse manager. And even see if you can get your preceptor to write a letter of recommendation to the nurse manager. Kelly did that for me, which was a huge help.

Perhaps more importantly, be teachable. Proverbs 16:18 says "Pride comes before destruction, and an arrogant spirit before a fall." Arrogance will kill you quickly and bring you down really fast. It's better to look stupid and to impress people than to act smart and important and be proven otherwise. The truth always comes out. Let people teach you. Be slow to be offended. Always smile and let your speech be gracious even when it's hard. Always say thank you. It will go well with you in the end if you do.

Nursing Process in Rehab/Clinical Management. Rehab nursing. Sigh. Again, if it's your niche, go for it. In the lecture portion of this class, we did learn some interesting things. Again though, it's one of those courses where you learn a lot of little details and facts so you can do well on the tests. You really do need to know the facts. You'll learn all about stroke and how it affects the body and the body's functions. Know what parts of the brain affect which functions. Stroke can be and often is devastating. In this class, you learn all about that—bladder and bowel dysfunction, personality changes, musculoskeletal disability, and swallowing problems. You also learn about traumatic brain injury and the repercussions of that. You learn about spinal cord injury. There was even a little piece where we learned about how to help these patients adapt sexually.

My instructor for this course was really in to it. She would act things out and even tell stories. It was obvious she liked the material, which helped a lot because she would deviate from just reading from the screen. I do recommend reading the textbook for this course. It's interesting stuff. And once again, you'll be grateful in this class that you paid attention and worked hard in A & P. That information will never go away. It'll make this class a little easier for you if you know your A&P.

One of our assignments for this class was very interesting and enlightening. Many of my peers found it to be somewhat disparaging, though. We were split into groups of two or three. Each person had to pretend to be handicapped for about six hours and their partner(s) were the helper(s). We could choose to be a paraplegic, hemiplegic, or quadriplegic, but whatever we chose, we had to play the part. We had to go out in a public place too…in a wheelchair. It was an interesting experience. Oh, and we had to wear an adult brief/diaper product and for a certain number of hours, the diaper had to be wet (we could choose to urinate ourselves or just put water in the diaper). Yes, eeewww. This project wasn't horrible, but it was very time consuming and difficult to coordinate a time to do it with the two other girls in my group. Anyhow, I've included the paper for you in the Appendix.

The clinical portion of this course wasn't too bad. As a matter of fact, I think it only lasted two weeks and was about six days total. We did have to do a case study. We followed one patient each during the whole time. I followed a very kind lady who'd had back surgery (a laminectomy) and was at the rehab center for physical and occupational therapy. Physical therapy (PT) and occupational therapy (OT) can be a real struggle for sick or physically disabled people, but it's neat to see their progress when they do stick it out. It was in fact, probably the most laid back clinical. We weren't allowed to pass meds, but we could assist PTs and others with their tasks. In this rotation, it was neat to see the thought processes behind the medications prescribed and given to these patients. It was neat to learn about, in the case of my patient, why the nurse should give her a muscle relaxant verses a narcotic before her PT sessions. Rehab nursing, in my humble opinion, is dry and dull compared to the field I'm currently in. My observation of the nurses in this facility was that they pretty much just pushed a cart all day and passed pills. It seemed a little robotic to me, but of course, that's just my observation over a two-week period. Perhaps there's more to it than that.

Community Health Nursing II. This was the sequel to

Community Health Nursing I that I talked about earlier. So, this semester we worked with the same group as we did last semester. This time, however, we took everything we had learned and all the information and data we had gathered from the previous semester on our group and we started working toward our well-defined goal. We wanted to improve the health status of our aggregate and we had, in writing, a clear definition of what that meant. We had clear steps and we developed a plan to get there. We spent a lot of time during this last busy semester of nursing school helping this group get healthier. We did little walks and exercises with them. At the end of the semester, we presented all of our data and results of how we had improved the health status of our aggregate by implementing some sort of program or teaching.

I can't locate the group paper we did, but we did alright with it. I remember that I was the final proofreader. I was trying so hard to get this paper done early, but some of my group members were waiting until the last minute to submit their portions, so it was a little annoying for me. The School of Nursing really made a big deal about this final presentation; I think they called it "Healthy People Presentations." We presented in front of a large audience, which consisted of the junior year nursing students and a lot of the faculty. I just remember sitting in the back tuning out once my group was finished. We had presented on May 1st and this was really one of the last things on my checklist before graduation, so I was kind of over it, as graduation was in 10 days and my wedding in 24.

Studies in Professional Nursing. It took some serious thinking for me to remember what this class was about. This course was worth two credits and we could take it either junior or senior year or during the summertime to get it over with. It was, in my opinion, another one of those silly things they made us do to graduate. I really don't think it was necessary. Anyhow, they gave us a list of different courses to choose from. One was about being environmentally friendly, one was about genetics in nursing, and there were a few others I can't recall. Each class just looked at a different topic that affects nursing or that nursing influences. I chose to take my elective senior year, the last semester. A lot of my peers took it sooner just so that they wouldn't have to think about it during the last semester before graduation. Each elective was entirely online. I know I chose the genetics course because I had already taken genetics for bio majors at the university, so I figured it would give me a head start. We did have to purchase some extra learning tool online so that we could have access to reading material that the instructor used for online questions. Uuuhh, it was a waste of time and it was one of those classes that you look at and wonder why education has to cost so much. We taught ourselves everything. We had to read the material and take quizzes and answer questions and do group discussions online about them. We even had to do a group paper. Again. Aaahhh! I don't know why the faculty had this obsession with group papers. I'd rather write five papers by myself than one with 10 group members.

Sadly, I can't even remember any of the details of what was learned in this class. I didn't retain anything past one week. What a joke.

Chapter 2: Surviving Nursing School

That basically sums up the nursing school curriculum that I went through. Hopefully it answered some questions for you about the courses you're looking at. At this point, I'd like to discuss some basic tips for not just getting through nursing school, but for actually doing well in it and enjoying it to the fullest (because I do believe that life is meant to be enjoyed).

I'd also like to add this: You can tell I had my frustrations with my undergraduate nursing curriculum. My university (and I think most universities do) had student opinion surveys at the end of each semester. I always made a conscious effort to fill them out because it allows professors and administrators to get student feedback. It's a chance to voice those frustrations in a positive way, which could possibly spark much needed changes. So, if you're going to complain about your nursing program, at least do it so that the right people hear you. Don't *just* write a book about it ☺.

1) Get enough sleep. I can't emphasize this enough. Your brain function, decision-making, and physical endurance are much more effective when you've had a good night's rest. It'll make you more productive, healthier, and a nicer person to be around.

2) Exercise. Yes, I've always moved around a lot. Being stationary is death. If you notice yourself constantly zoning out while trying to study for an exam or if you're lacking motivation or focus, just take a break and go outside and walk around the block. Fresh air does a lot of good. Get your blood moving and flowing to your brain. Also, exercise will help you sleep at night. It's all around great for you. I could go into a long spiel here but I'm trying to resist. Exercise fights depression, keeps your hormones in balance, and makes you feel good. In the words of Nike, just do it.

3) Eat right. Food is the best preventative maintenance and it is the all-natural medicine. Your body will thank you. A banana and some scrambled eggs and nuts/oatmeal will do you a whole lot more good before an exam than a sugary donut and an energy

drink. When you're stressed, don't reach for food to comfort you. It'll cause problems if it becomes a habit. Also, if you don't know how to read a nutrition label, what better time to learn than in nursing school? Understand how many calories your body needs and choose them wisely. Understand the importance of fat in your diet. It's not the enemy people make it out to be. Understand fiber, the glycemic index, and sugar. Know about protein. You should get this info from your time in A & P. Again, pay attention in that class. It is worthwhile. Know why an apple is a better choice than a Slurpee. Trust me. When you're nice to your body, it'll be nice to you.

Also, eating right is one of the best things you can do to prevent weight gain while in school. Many of my peers packed on 10-15 pounds (which may not sound like a lot, but 15 pounds of fat is hard to take off) while in the nursing program. I didn't gain a pound because I'm pretty good at stress management. Prioritizing, eating right, sleeping, and exercising all work together in the effort to not gain weight while in school. Just remember balance.

One of my greatest pet peeves is the fact that health care workers, nurses in particular, are some of the unhealthiest people I know. Many of them are overweight, sleep deprived, and stressed out. What's worse is some smoke! How can you counsel someone into a state of health when you're a train wreck yourself?!

4) Find a solid support system. You're going to consider quitting nursing school at some point. And you will see all your friends out and about doing fun things while you're stuck inside the library studying. You'll get a bad grade and think you're a failure. You'll have a mean clinical instructor who will make you cry. Hard times will come. Get a solid person you can count on to cheer you up and tell you the truth and remind you of why you're doing this. If you're married, it should be your spouse. If you're not married, maybe your greatest support system is your parents, an uncle or aunt, a co-worker, a classmate, a friend from church, or a neighbor. Find a solid person you can go to for encouragement. Make sure it's someone who knows you well so that he or she will be honest with you. Proverbs 27:9b – "The sweetness of a friend is better than self-counsel."

Also, I encourage everyone to find a best friend at school. By best friend, I really just mean a trustworthy peer that you can count on for back-up. Say all hell breaks loose in your life the week before finals and you need someone to e-mail you the notes from class and to fill you in on important details about the upcoming final for critical care. Find somebody who's got your back. Get that person's number and e-mail too. And it's not somebody that can cut you slack or someone that you can pester or have do your work for you (that's called cheating), but someone you can go to for help if something really is wrong and you need back-up. Make sure this person has a decent track record before you hire them as your go-to during a bad time. Unfortunately, some people don't have their stuff together. And sadly, some people will intentionally mislead you. I remember a classmate from my first semester at the university. We took a basic English writing course together. She had asked me for my username and log in to Blackboard where we submitted papers and saw our grades because she had some issue and couldn't access her account. That girl was nuts. I hardly even knew her. No, I wasn't going to give her access to the account through which she could pay bills, e-mail instructors, see my grades and submit "my" assignments. Ludicrous. Again, just think it through when it comes to trusting people.

5) Keep the end in mind. Constantly and as often as necessary,

remind yourself of why you chose nursing. Remind yourself of why you're taking the path you're taking. Maybe it's to get a better job where you'll make more money; maybe you really want to help people; maybe this is the first step in your endeavor to land your dream job as a nurse midwife or a family nurse practitioner; maybe you're a single mom or dad who's doing it for your kids. Whatever the reason (and most nurses I know went into this profession for a good reason), remind yourself of it frequently. It'll help to get you through. Also, remind yourself that you want to be competent on the job, so anything and everything you can learn in school is usually to your benefit.

6) Don't stress (over the little things). A little bit of stress isn't so bad. But, three years worth of anxiety and worry is really horrible for you. It sucks you dry of creativity and clear thinking. It robs you of your joy. How, you might ask, am I supposed to not stress in a seemingly stressful major? Honestly, prepare. As I discussed in the Introduction ("How to do Well in Your Pre-Requisites"), organize with a planner. It's not a bad idea to go over your planner with your school buddy and make sure you guys didn't overlook any important dates.

7) Learn to manage your time wisely. I could have tacked this on to the last paragraph. Perhaps the greatest equalizer of human beings is time. We are all given 60 minutes in an hour; we're each given 24 hours in one day; we're each given seven days in one week. Of course, lifespan varies. Spend your time wisely. Refer back to the final semester of senior year that I talked about earlier. For me, the first part of that semester was not so crazy because I was not in rehab class yet and I was not in my preceptorship yet. Instead of twiddling my thumbs and doing nothing, I looked way ahead in my planner. I could see that for the silly "Studies in Professional Nursing" class, I had upcoming assignments. For another course, "Leadership, Management, and Professional Development" (the writing course), I knew there was an important paper due a few weeks out. I went ahead and spent this chill time knocking all those assignments out.

In the category of time management, understand what is important to you. Nursing school (and school in general) will require you to sacrifice something. You may find it difficult to work 40 hours a week and go to school full-time. Figure out if there's a way you can creatively cut down on the number of hours you need to work while in school (without having to borrow money). For example, do you really need to stop at Starbucks while in route to school in order to purchase a $5 specialty coffee drink when you could just get a container of Maxwell House coffee from Costco for $8 and brew 320 cups of java at home? That saves money, and hence, could mean you can work a little less. Or, if you're a youngin' and your parents are up for it, live at home. Don't live on campus if you don't have to. That'll save you, what, $10,000/year? Stow your car away during the week and walk to school or ride your bike to save in gas. Or carpool. Buy used books. Reuse binders. Take care of what you do have. Wear your shoes for more than a year. Shop at the thrift store if you "need" a new outfit. Use the same cell phone for more than a month. I could go on and on about this, but simplify your life as much as possible while you're in school.

I encourage people to really balance the whole work-school life. Working while in school can be a good thing and even helps some people to do better in school, but it can also make doing well academically very difficult. If you're fortunate enough to have supportive parents or whoever (fill in the blank), or if you're on some sort of scholarship, take that funding seriously and don't work if you don't have to. I worked just one shift a week at the nursing home as a nurse aide and was raking in $135 every two weeks. This was good for me because it reminded me of why I was in nursing school and what I'd be stuck doing the rest of my life if I didn't get through it (CNA work is rough!). It also gave me a slight sense of independence and self-pride knowing that I could afford to put gas in my car and buy myself a sandwich if I wanted. I also just wanted to show my parents that I was grateful for their assistance and that I wasn't a complete moocher, although they never made me work by any means; they actually encouraged me not to. If you must work, I recommend working in some sort of health care job or area that you're going to be working in upon graduating. It helps to build your experience and offers some great networking opportunities. Volunteering is great, but I wouldn't overdo it. You're a college student and tuition is not cheap. If you're going to help somebody, get paid for it. I know that sounds selfish, but really, when you're in school, your time matters. And often, you need time more than money.

Also, when it comes to time management, I want to point

something out in terms of studying. When you're preparing for an exam, if there's some chunk of test material that you already know really well, don't spend your time studying that and reviewing it ad nauseam. Study what you don't know. Focus your efforts there. My high school Bible teacher taught me this. Don't waste your time.

Do your work at the time that's best for you. I can't tell you when that is. For me, it's morning. That's when I'm sharpest. I'd rather knock out my important schoolwork in the morning (between 8 and noon) and then spend my afternoon doing what I want. Focus. It's hard but you can do it. On the same note, if you're completely exhausted and trying to study information late at night, stop. Go to bed, get some rest, and wake up and get some focused, sharp studying in for just 30 minutes in the morning. It's better than staring aimlessly at your notes for two hours at night when you're not going to retain anything. Go to sleep. Spend your time wisely.

8) Respect people. This may sound like a silly thing to say. But really, you'd be surprised at how much of a challenge it can be at times. You'll meet people that you think are complete idiots and

you'll wonder how they even got in to college. You'll wonder how people can be so close-minded or even how they can be so open-minded. Be kind to people and listen to what they have to say. You don't have to agree. If nothing else, just state back to them what they told you. Learn people's names. Write them down. Remember people. You'll run into some "important" folks while in school. Try as best as you can to get along with everyone, especially faculty. You never know when you'll need to get a letter of recommendation from one of them. They're great resources, so try to get on their good side. Most importantly, they're people, and people in general are worth relationships. Also, try to meet managers and other nurses where you do clinicals. Remember, it's great networking and it could help you down the road.

Be nice and polite. It never fails. Always take the high road. Be slow to get offended. If you're emotional, angry, frustrated, offended, fill in the blank—just play it safe and say nothing. It's much harder to mess up that way. Romans 13:17-19 says: "Do not repay anyone evil for evil. Try to do what is honorable in everyone's eyes. If possible, on your part, live at peace with everyone. Friends, do not avenge yourselves; instead, leave room for His wrath. For it is written: Vengeance belongs to Me; I will repay, says the Lord." Control yourself and things will work out.

Chapter 3: The NCLEX

If only you could go through nursing school, get your degree, and then start working. It's not quite that simple. Since you are planning to go into a field where people's lives will be in your hands, you have to jump through an extra hoop before you can start working. This major hoop is called the NCLEX. It stands for National Council Licensure Exam. Passing the NCLEX is how you get licensed. Without passing it, you are not licensed and thus cannot practice nursing. Now, some places will hire you before you've passed the NCLEX, but you must pass it within a certain period of being hired, like within 90 days or within six months. That was my situation. I graduated May 11th and took the NCLEX on June 25th. I started working on June 17th.

Take the NCLEX seriously. Fortunately, my nursing

program prided itself on its high pass rate for the NCLEX. I think it was something like 98% when I was there. That's a major factor as to whether or not your school gets accredited. My university's curriculum is all geared toward students being able to pass this exam. The reason the school was so focused on students passing it is because that's what really matters. You can have a 4.0 GPA, but if you can't pass that test, guess what, you can't work as a nurse. The NCLEX proves that you are competent and know at least the bare minimum to safely practice as a registered nurse.

The NCLEX is like your final of finals. It is cumulative and covers everything you learned throughout nursing school. That can sound a bit overwhelming. Relax. There are plenty of companies out there that offer review courses, kind of like how there are review courses for kids wanting to take the MCAT for medical school. I highly recommend taking one of these courses. I took the one offered called the HURST Review. Dr. Winn set it up at the school about a week after we graduated. It cost some money; I want to say it was like $300 or so. Richard was a sweetheart and knew our future really depended on me passing the test, so he encouraged me to take it and he even paid for it. Now, this class was the week before my wedding, so I had a lot of things on my mind, but I knew it was important. It only lasted for a few hours of the day, like from 8-12 or 8-2, something like that. They handed us this decent-sized manual and told us that was all we needed to know for the NCLEX. The book was set up by systems/areas of nursing. It was fill-in-the blank and we had an instructor who would lecture and fill in the blanks as he talked. If you're someone who learns that way, great. The course also gave you access to different videos and lectures online. You could also do NCLEX review questions online too. A lot of helpful hints are given in this course. I have to be careful here because I can get in trouble if I say too much about the HURST review. You can get into some serious trouble if you give that booklet away to someone who didn't pay for it or if you spill too much info about the class. Anyhow, HURST review is considered a course on content review, whereas the Kaplan course, I was told, is more of a strategy course in which you're given info on how to answer the NCLEX questions. I chose HURST because I knew that there would be a lot of information on the exam. If I had good test-taking strategies but didn't know content, what good would that be? And, in nursing school, Dr. Winn and a few other instructors gave us some helpful hints on how to answer those difficult strategy questions where every answer seemed right. Most important to me was the content review.

Looking back, I think the HURST review was well worth the money. The NCLEX costs close to $300 to take. You don't want to take it twice. I prepped and reviewed that book that they gave us over and over and over again. I took practice quizzes and even ordered from Amazon the book *The NCLEX, Made Incredibly Easy*. Those were my two major study tools. I think maybe once or twice I cracked open my Med-Surge textbook to read a few things in-depth. But it's true, that if you know your basic facts of A & P and you understand physiology, you can figure things out. And the majority of the NCLEX is Med-Surge. Specialty areas are included on it, though. So again, that's why I stuck to that manual they gave us in the HURST review. The lady who designed the course swore that if we knew that content in the manual by heart, we'd pass the first time. So I took her word for it. It's a heck of a lot easier to study 300 pages of material as opposed to thousands. And I highly recommend taking as many practice quizzes as you can. And read the feedback. Understand what the NCLEX questions are going to look like. The more practice you can get, the better.

I started studying for the NCLEX once Richard and I got back from our honeymoon. I gave myself a solid two weeks of focused study time. My work schedule wasn't crazy yet, so I spent my time at home reading through that manual over and over again. When that got old, I'd switch to the NCLEX Made Easy book. Then I'd take the quizzes. I didn't kill myself, but I did put in a few solid hours of studying each morning. Again, study when you're the sharpest. If I felt myself dozing off, I'd take a break or call it good for the day and then go out and do something else. But you do need to study appropriately for this exam.

Your instructor (for us, it was Dr. Winn) should go over how to sign up for the NCLEX. You have to get your official transcript after graduation and mail that to the state board of nursing once you graduate. They have to do some correspondence and send you a ticket to test. Then you can go on the website and register for the NCLEX in your area. I chose to take it June 25th because it was after the wedding and honeymoon hype were over. Don't schedule this exam during some life-changing event, like the day after your baby is due or the morning of your wedding day or even the day that your dog has surgery. Try, as much as you can, to devote a whole day to this test. It can be quite anxiety-producing, so make it its own thing. I slept well the night before and didn't cram for it. I scheduled it at 8 am. Richard made me a fantastic breakfast—coffee, water, scrambled eggs, and oatmeal with fruit. I devoured that and left the house with plenty of time to get there. They won't let you carry anything into that test; I don't even think I could take water. When they go over the rules in that place, make sure you follow them. Don't get kicked out for something stupid like bringing your cell phone in. Also, before you even leave your house, make sure you have that sheet of paper that says you are allowed to take the test. I almost forgot mine.

    I sat down in a cubicle-like place with the computer in front of me. I remember early into the test, I got this horrendous headache. And I don't get those often. Then my vision started acting funky and it was hard for me to read the screen. The proctor told me it couldn't be adjusted. I continued and pushed through. I remember getting a lot of those multiple-multiple questions, also called the alternate-format questions where you have to "select all that apply." I figured this was a good thing, because it meant I was getting the higher-level questions, which meant things were going well. I was so grateful when, after I hit "Submit" after the 75th question, the test ended. I had heard from others who had taken the test with just 75 questions, that close to all of them had passed. However, I had also heard that you could fail if you only got 75 questions. The test is weird. Some people pass with 200 + questions, while others fail with only 75. I think you have to reach some special mark before it turns off. I was so relieved just when the thing was over, and I felt pretty confident.

When I walked out, I called Richard and told him it was over. Then I went over to the mall and saw my mom (where she worked) and got a pretzel to eat. My headache started resolving. Later in the afternoon, I tried the trick where you try to sign up again to take the NCLEX. If the phone or computer doesn't let you, it supposedly means you passed. You don't know for sure that you passed, though, until you can go online and/or call the state board and get your RN license number. Then it's official. I think this came for me the following day. Talk about a weight being lifted.

I would assume the NCLEX is like labor for a mother-to-be.

The more prepared you are, the better.

Part 2: On the Job

Prologue

My nursing career started out as below stated. I hadn't planned to include nursing home stories in this book, but I later realized that they're too good to leave out. At age 21, the summer before nursing school began, I started working at a nursing home. This place had four units, and each room housed two patients. It was a pretty large facility. Some of the people who lived there had chronic illnesses or were extremely disabled because of sickness and thus needed 24/7 care. Other patients were there for six weeks or so to get focused rehabilitation each day through physical therapy and occupational therapy.

I was naïve and as full of life as could be. People would call me "little girl" and "smiley" (some of the nicer titles I've been given in this profession). I was a shining star and gosh-darned determined to make the world a better place. It was my first day on the job as a certified nursing assistant (CNA) and I was ready to conquer the world. I was prepared to be a light in a dark place—a nursing home.

I arrived in my neon green scrub top, black scrub pants, and cushy snow-white nursing shoes. My hair was long and straightened, pulled back into a pony tail. I made my way into that one-story brick building on a pretty morning in May, 6:45 am, 15 minutes before the shift started. I swiped my badge, took a left, and made my way down the hall, passing several patient's rooms along the way. "Nuuuuurrrrsssssee!!!" I heard one person shout. A thin white woman with short curly brown hair and bright red lipstick sat in her wheelchair on the side of the hallway. She was one of the nursing home patients, and kindly smiled at me as I walked by. Taking care of people in need was going to be great.

"*Ohhhhh mmmmyyyy woooorrrrddd,*" I thought to myself as I continued down the hall. "They must have had a sewer line break somewhere nearby." Then I noticed a woman in scrubs walk out of a room. She was carrying three plastic bags full of paper-like materials. There was some sort of brown sludge in the bags too. "Hmmm, I guess she cleaned it up." I then made my way behind the nurses station to the break area for the morning pow-wow. I was so excited.

When I got to the break room, I spotted several other women sitting there in scrubs. The break room was small. Two of the women sat on the bench. One lady, who was very strong-looking, had her back to the door. I stood just inside the doorway and noticed all of their chatter stop. All of them but the one in the chair looked at me. I noticed two other workers file in. I smiled. "Hi everyone, my name's Rebecca. Today's my first day and I'm really happy to meet you guys. I'm looking forward to learning from you all." With my teeth-showing smile still on my face, I saw the woman in the chair turn around to face me. She had large hands and a tired face. She had long eyelashes and her eyes were outlined with thick eyeliner. Her bright pink studded earrings glowed against her dark earlobes. She looked at me with an expressionless face. She opened her mouth. "Well REEEEeeebecca, welcome to helllll."

Chapter 4: The CNA Experience

The Beginning. I spent a few weeks in orientation, in which I worked alongside a more experienced nurse aide. Early on in my endeavor as a CNA, one co-worker showed me how she cleaned up an incontinent patient who was in the bed. "You just roll 'em back and forth. Use these wipes. Roll the dirty diaper under this way. Tuck the new diaper down here. Roll 'em back this way, and then patch the diaper up with the tabs." It irked me that she kept referring to incontinent briefs as "diapers." I had been taught in my CNA course to call them "peri pads" or "briefs" because the term diaper was disparaging. The poor patient was as stiff as a board. She was helpless as my co-worker rolled her back and forth in the bed. "Yep, it's just a job," my co-worker said as we walked out of the room holding the trash bag of soiled undergarments and dirty wipes.

"Go ahead. She dirty," my supervising co-worker said to me as we stood just inside a patient's room staring into the bed. As we got closer, I thought I was going to vomit. It was the most putrid thing I'd ever smelled. I tried not to breathe through my nose. "Hi, we're here to help get you cleaned up," I said softly and with an attempted smile, trying to hide the fact that I wanted to vomit due to the odor coming from the patient I was about to help. The frail woman stared back at me. I slowly pulled the sheet back from her body. Gulp. There was a large puddle of dark black liquid stool all around her. I tried to suppress my disgust. I worked to roll the patient to her side while talking to her gently. She was heavy. "I'm cleaning you up now," I told her gently. As I worked, I got confused as to how to put the clean brief on. "Carla, will you help me," I asked my co-worker who was supervising. She came and gave me a hand and we finished our task. Stool was everywhere.

I quickly realized in this job that the most important thing was making sure all the patients assigned to me were clean and dry, meaning that they'd had proper and frequent incontinence care (making sure they weren't sitting in their urine and feces). One day

I was written up by my supervisor because I'd left a patient up in her chair. When the shift came on after me and the patient was put back in bed, she was completely soiled. How could I get written up for that? There was no way I could have had time to clean that patient again before my shift ended. She was the first one I'd gotten up in the morning. It took me eight hours to go through just one round of helping all my patients. Again, I worked the first shift, 7am-3pm and so I was responsible for providing all morning ADLs (activities of daily living—oral hygiene (brushing teeth), bathing, incontinence care, dressing, etc.), morning vital signs, getting patients up out of bed and into the dining hall, and feeding breakfast and lunch to those who could not feed themselves. I normally had eight to 12 patients to care for each shift. Most of the patients were completely helpless and many of them were more than twice my weight.

    I felt defeated very early on, especially when it came to documenting all of my work. There was simply not enough time, or manpower, to do all the things required for all of these patients. I had to choose between brushing their teeth, providing incontinence care, bathing, feeding, and getting them up out of bed for the day. There was not enough time to do it all! And I hated having to document that I hadn't brushed someone's teeth or hadn't given him a drink in four hours. I wasn't going to lie and chart something I didn't do. I quickly learned to adapt and focus on the most important things –incontinence care and getting up the patients who were supposed to be up. I realized most of the patients at that nursing home had probably not had their teeth/gums cleaned in years.

One morning I was making rounds to get vital signs on my patients to give to the nurses before their med pass. I entered one patient's dark room. He was sleeping. The TV was still on from the night before. "Hi Mr. Ogden, I'm Rebecca. I'm just here to get your vital signs," I whispered very softly. I proceeded to put the blood pressure cuff on his arm. "What the fu*k are you doing?!! Get the he*l out of here! What the fu*k!!!" he yelled as his eyes opened. "I'm sorry to disturb you, Mr. Ogden, it's just that it's time for morning vitals," I replied. "I don't give a sh*t!" he stammered back. "I get up first and *then* they take my vital signs." He was a relatively younger patient. He was paralyzed from the waist down. He was awake and so I offered to help him get up and he was agreeable to that. After spending some significant time bathing him and picking out his particular outfit, it was time to get him out of bed. He was going to require the hoyer lift, an electronic piece of equipment that acted sort of as a hammock that lifted patients out of their bed and into a chair or vice versa. All hoyer lift transfers require two staff members. "I'll be back," I said.

    I walked quickly down the hall and into the break room to look for help. "Hey guys, can I get a hand getting Mr. Ogden up? I'm gonna grab the hoyer lift now." "Why you gettin him up?" was the response. "*Umm, because it's my job,*" I thought in my head. I replied, "It's time for him to get up and he wants to get up." The ladies in the break room were very reluctant to move, as it was still early in the shift. They staggered and so eventually I got the help of a nurse who was wondering why the other aides didn't help me. I didn't explain that to her in depth because I didn't want to get my co-workers in trouble. We got Mr. Ogden up in his electric wheelchair. He and I got along pretty well from then on. He just liked things a certain way.

    It was time to go into Room 31. The patient in the A bed

(closest to the door) was already up. I proceeded to help the patient in the B bed. "Hi, Mr. Solomon, my name's Rebecca. I'm a nurse aide. I'm here to help you with your bath and to help you get up for the day." I smiled and looked at him. He smiled back, but only the left side of his face moved. He was sitting up in the bed, shirtless, with a sheet pulled up to his waist. He was a Caucasian man, in his 50s. He wore glasses. I looked around and noticed crumbs all over his bed. There was an open drawer protruding from his nightstand, where there were bags of candies and chips.

"Becky," he murmured, "you're really pretty." "Well thanks," I replied. I grabbed some washcloths and towels and a basin of water and proceeded to bathe him. His eyes stared at me and when I looked at him, he smiled back. He asked me about my age, my boyfriend, my (non-existent) children, and how long I'd worked there. Like a fool, I went into detail in answering every question he asked me. I thought Mr. Solomon was kind. He told me not to call him mister and not to call him sir because it made him feel old. So I started calling him by his first name—Dan.

At first, Dan was one of my favorite patients to care for. He shared with me some of his story and how he'd ended up in the nursing home. He had a seizure disorder that kept him from working. He'd also suffered a stroke at one point and lost use of his entire right side. He got around well, though, in his motorized wheelchair. Dan would always say he was happy to see me at work.

One day Dan got a new roommate who I also was very fond of. His name was Mr. C. Turns out I'd gone to high school with a kid whose family he had a connection to. Mr. C had a very soft voice. He was a white man with orange hair. He loved Jesus. And bicycles. I would often help him bathe, get dressed, and get up. He took longer to help because he had Parkinson's disease. I'd often get Dan up first so he could get on with his day and then I'd help Mr. C. One day I noticed Dan and Mr. C in the hallway together. Dan was in front, sitting in his electric wheelchair. I heard "Hang on, Clyde (referring to Mr. C)." I walked closer and noticed that Mr. C has his arms stretched out. He was in his non-electric wheelchair hanging on to the back of Dan's for a ride. Just imagine two dudes in their 50s and 60s pulling this stunt. I thought it was genius but one of the nurses quickly broke up their fun.

One day while bathing Mr. C, he started talking about Dan.

"You know, Rebecca, sometimes at night Dan watches things on TV that are bad. I want him to know Jesus." Mr. C was like a missionary. His physical strength was waning, but his heart and compassion were so strong. During my time at the nursing home, I saw his condition steadily decline. He developed severe dysphagia (difficulty swallowing). Ultimately this led to a pneumonia. He was moved to an isolation room because his respiratory condition and immune system were so weak. I remember helping him one day. His face was pale and he could hardly speak. He wanted to express something but couldn't say it. "Mr. C, I have to move on to help some other folks now." I can still see his eyes looking into mine as I walked out of his room. He laid in the bed, hardly able to move. Drool poured out of his mouth even though I'd just used the oral suction device on him. "I'll see you later, Mr. C." But I didn't. I knew he was in bad shape. I heard shortly thereafter at work that he had passed away.

Creeper. Dan and I reminisced about Mr. C and how it was too bad that he was gone. One day I helped bathe Dan. His eyes watched me as I rubbed the damp washcloth over his chest. "Becky," he said. "Can I touch your breast?" *Did I hear that* *right?*", I thought. "No," I said firmly but not in a harsh tone. I proceeded to finish the task at hand. The following day, Dan asked if I'd told anyone what he'd asked me. I told him no. I continued through the weeks and months providing care for Dan. Some of his other remarks ("Nice legs," "If you were my woman, I'd run my fingers through your hair") finally became eerie enough that I woke up to them. I never addressed him but began to separate myself from him by asking for a change in my patient assignment. One day, he rode up to me in his wheelchair and asked me if I didn't like him anymore. The whole thing was very awkward and I sort of ran from it like a coward. He was creepy. Even to this day, I'll sometimes have nightmares of him chasing me in his wheelchair. When I left that job, I didn't say goodbye to him. I did care about Dan as a person, though. I pitied him in many ways because of his condition, so I wanted to be his friend. He stepped over the line and I should have shot it down sooner. He wanted a friend. I was creeped out and didn't really know the right way to handle the situation, so I just ran from it.

    There was another creeper story that occurred after I had been at the nursing home a little while and had a little bit of experience. It involved an overweight patient, in his 40s, who needed a lot of assistance. I went into his room and introduced myself. "Ohhhh heeeyyy, you pretty thing is gonna clean me up?" was his response to my introduction. "I'm gonna run some water and get some towels, alright." As I bathed him and got closer to his groin area, he became very disrespectful. "Oooo, yeah, you gonna clean up daddy down there?" "Mr. Alfred, you need to stop that right now. Continue on and I'll walk right out of here and leave you in your mess. Stop." "Huuhh, I'm gonna tell your manager that you're disrespecting me," was his reply. It was late in the shift and I did not care about much. I was tired. "Go ahead; I'm just trying to do my job, Mr. Alfred, and you're being inappropriate" is what I told him. He finally piped down and I was able to finish getting him cleaned.

One more story on female CNA exploitation/sexual nuisance/harassment – A much older, big boned Caucasian man named Charles seemed to have some suppressed emotions that decided to come out in his older age. He made eye contact with me the entire time I worked bathing him and getting him dressed. He was really difficult to move; he was rigid and thick. He could see how hard it was for someone my size to turn him back and forth in the bed trying to get his clothes on. He just looked at me with a smirk on his face the whole time, as if the whole experience was pleasurable for him. It was very uncomfortable for me, just trying to work. "How many babies you got?," he would ask me almost daily. When I was new my answer was "none." Then I started to have fun and one day told him "96" when he asked. He seemed to know I was joking. "What color are your panties?" he asked me another time. I believe I just ignored him. My husband down the road said I should have replied with "white with a brown streak in the middle." Eeeewww. What was really odd was meeting Charles' sons when they would come to visit. It was just weird.

There was a woman I cared for who was very contracted (many of her joints were locked in a flexed position). She was bedridden and the most she could really do for herself was feed herself. Her legs were locked in a bent position and any movement was painful. She was very kind, though, and I really felt sorry for her, so I tried to spend extra time helping her. I made it a point to brush her teeth, since they were stained and I knew she couldn't do it herself. I bathed her with care. Incontinence care was very difficult due to her contractures. She would ask me to put in the DVD of her favorite movie. As I did so, I would see pictures on her wall behind the TV of a young couple on some tropical beach. She told me that it was her and her husband. All the times I helped that woman I never saw her husband. I thought of the life she once lived, young and healthy, able to move. Now she couldn't even get out of bed. It was tragic to me. She later died of respiratory failure.

Another man was in a similar position. He was probably in his late 40s, early 50s and had been electrocuted. He was bedridden and totally dependent. Whenever I helped him, I wondered when the last time was that he'd been outside or had his teeth brushed. He was cognizant enough to nod his head. One Saturday I actually had some extra time. After bathing him and brushing his teeth, I asked if he'd like to go outside. He nodded yes. So, I used the hoyer lift and got him into his mobile recliner chair. It was a beautiful day. I wheeled him out to where there was a wooden bridge over a small creek near the parking lot. We sat there for a few minutes in the sun. It was lovely.

One woman was young, probably early 30s. She was a complete vegetable other than the fact she could open her eyes.

She had to be fed through a tube, was incontinent, couldn't talk, couldn't walk. Her life was lying in a bed at the end of the hall. The story I'd heard was that something went wrong with an epidural she received during childbirth. The most contact she had with the outside world was looking out the window and hearing whatever someone put on her TV. I didn't even know for sure if she could still hear or comprehend things, but whenever I went in to clean her up, I would tell her the date and what the weather was like outside. I'd tell her about current events. The only person I ever saw visit her was her sister.

The most depressing floor was called the trach unit. Patients there had often sustained really bad strokes and could no longer breathe for themselves or swallow; some had end-stage COPD. Many of them seemed to be on death's doorstep. Bathing and turning them was very difficult because most of them were entirely helpless. I remember thinking to myself that I'd rather just die than be in their shoes.

One of these patients I cared for was a Hispanic woman who'd sustained a pretty bad stroke. She was 100% dependent on others for care. As a new aide, I was in her room cleaning her up one day. I committed the cardinal sin: I had the patient turned onto her left side; when I moved to the right side of the bed, I did not put the railing up on the side she was laying on. The bed was up at my torso level. I was on the right side of the bed preparing to help her when I saw body roll and then there she went. Thump. My patient had just fallen off the bed.

Ah, crap! Did that just happen?! I panicked internally. *I hope she's not hurt! What if she hit her head?"* I was afraid to move around to the other side to look at her, afraid she'd hit her head and was unconscious. I was sure to lose my job for this. Her family would probably kill me when they found out about it. I went to the other side of the bed and looked down at my naked patient. There was no blood anywhere. She was breathing and looked like her normal self; just, on the floor, not in the bed. I told her I'd get some help and we'd get her up. I quickly moved down the hall to the nurses station. "Mrs. Berneger is on the floor," I said to some of my co-workers at the front desk. "What?!!" Several of them stood up and took off with me down the hall toward her room. We recruited a few others along the way. Of course, I had to explain what happened and I did feel like a complete ignoramus. I really felt bad for Mrs. Berneger too. I'm sure she'd cuss me out if she could talk. Fortunately, she was okay. We all worked together and used the hoyer lift to get her back in the bed. I never repeated that mistake since. Always put your side rails up if you're going to work on the opposite side of the bed that the patient is lying on.

If I were ever in the position of many of these nursing home patients, I know what I would want someone to do for me: be gentle, keep my bottom clean, brush my teeth, give me water, and take me outside. That's what I tried to do for them. Many of them were in such terrible shape. I learned that health is wealth. Many of them lived my worst nightmare each day—paralyzed, not able to talk or do anything independently, fully reliant on others for everything. I've always heard that it's not good to sympathize with people. Empathy is superior, at least that's what I learned in psychology class and many nursing classes. But I couldn't help it. I hadn't walked in these patient's shoes, although I did try to put myself there at times. My heart truly ached for many of them, especially the ones who had tasted freedom and independence at some point but had it revoked. Like the woman with all the contractures who could barely move. From her bed each day, she had to stare at the picture of her and her husband (probably honeymooning) on some tropical beach. She had tasted life, and now her life was confined to a bed. To me, it's one of the saddest things. Not being able to run, to see, to brush your own teeth, to wipe your own butt, reposition yourself, to go outside on a whim, to spend holidays in the cozy homes of your loved ones. If anything, being a CNA taught me to embrace life all the more. To really live it.

Dementia. Dementia, as sad as it is, I have to say was comical at times at the nursing home. There was a patient who didn't seem that old to me; he was probably in his 50s. He was a nice guy. I was completely fooled by him at first. He was agreeable to taking his own showers, brushing his teeth, and everything. One day I saw him walking down the hall. He had his long, collared shirt on, his gray sweatpants, baseball cap, and sneakers. "Hey, Mr. Brian, what are you up to?," I asked him. He replied back quietly (his usual tone), "Oh, there's a baseball game today that I've gotta get to." "Well, have fun." He continued down the hall. I realized later this man was very off. I'd find him at times sitting uninvited in other patient's rooms. He would talk about his plans to go places. One day, he kept on walking down the hall and managed to break out of the nursing home. Sirens and alarms sounded and I heard a nurse shout, "Oh no, it's Mr. Brian!" Several workers took off after him. He had gotten out to the main road outside the nursing home. Fortunately, his ankle bracelet was working and he was brought back safely. The man had some pretty bad dementia, but to a stranger, it seemed he was totally with it.

Ms. Reef was a character too. She was a very sweet African American patient. She wore her thick hair in a ponytail. I would help her get bathed, dressed, and up for the mornings. She did not like having her teeth brushed or her private areas cleaned. I got her up to the sink, where she saw herself in the mirror. "That looks just like me," she said and smiled widely. She had a soft voice and a gentle demeanor. When I'd help her, she'd start talking about random people and things. "He told me he wasn't gonna be at church." "Oh, are you talking about Mr. Parker?" I said back. "Yes, he told me he wasn't gonna be there." I'd make up lines, "Well, I heard he's getting married." "He's getting married?" she said back. It was so funny. We would have completely futile conversations but somehow I felt a sweet bond with this lady. She was so sweet, though, and I think she liked having someone to talk with. I'd find her at times in empty patients' rooms sitting in a chair in the dark talking to herself.

Wounds. Wound care was quite eye-opening at the nursing home. I didn't get to do the wound care as an aide, but I did help the nurses. To date, it is this nursing home patient who gets the award for the worst wound I've ever seen. He was a thin man in his 50s. His face always looked like it was in agony. The man had bipolar disease, multiple myeloma (a type of blood cell cancer), and HIV. As he lay in the bed, I helped to roll him onto his left side. My jaw dropped. There was a gaping hole at the base of his spine. The wound was a little bigger round than a large grapefruit. Some of the tissue in the wound was pink; there wasn't much blood. The most disturbing thing was that there was white matter inside that wound. As I stuck my face closer, I realized what it was. Bone. The pressure wound was so bad it had eroded all of his skin, subcutaneous fat (what little there was), and muscle. I was looking at his bare lumbar vertebrae. It was the worst wound I've ever seen.

Poop. If you can't handle poop (bowel movements,

excrement, feces, stool) do not go into nursing, especially not CNA work. Cleaning it is a big part of the job. One morning one of the nurses walked out of a room neglecting to inform me that she'd given a severely constipated patient an enema. I went into the room. It was on her top sheet. It was on the side of the bed. It was on the floor. This particular patient was also very contracted and difficult to move. It took some serious work, lots of wet wipes, towels and washcloths, and new linens. The stuff was everywhere and she was difficult to clean because her legs were basically locked together. Eventually, I got her all cleaned up and I know she felt better. Peppermint oil is a phenomenal thing. It's the best odor eliminator I've encountered. Keep it handy. Just a little of it goes a long way.

  I was working the 3-11PM shift. It was time to check on Ms. Mao as part of my last rounds for the evening. *Hmmm, she'll definitely need to be changed*, I thought, as I entered her dark room. It smelled like stool. The closer I got to the bed and to her, the more I smelled it. I turned on the dim light. I proceeded to remove her brief. Upon opening it, I saw that it was dry. There was a small streak in the back of it. *"Well, maybe she just has some bad gas.*" I patched the brief back up and prepared to leave her room when I noticed her hands. Her fingernails had brown residue under them. I thought maybe it was food. But a closer look revealed otherwise. There were a few brown streaks on her sheet as well. I looked around. *"So strange,"* I thought. As I turned around, I saw her bed table (a long wooden table on wheels; it can reach across the patient's bed) to the side. There it was. A small mound. Several formed brown pieces stacked on top of one another. I turned my attention to cleaning off the table.

I was helping a confused patient who was on isolation for C-diff (again, C-diff is infectious diarrhea; it usually results from intense antibiotic use. It has a very distinct odor and presentation). I proceeded to provide care for this woman, who had good use of her arms and legs. As I helped her, she pulled her hands out from under the sheet. They were covered in brown stuff. "What pretty hair you have," she said as she moved her hands toward my head, too close for comfort. "Let's clean those hands off," I said gently. That could've been bad.

Closing. I know that some of these CNA stories are scary. Looking back, I'm glad I worked as a CNA. I highly encourage anyone thinking about nursing to be an aide first. The backbreaking work you'll do as a nursing assistant will not disappear when you become an RN. If anything, having CNA skills will make you a better nurse. Spending some time as an aide will also give you a taste of what nursing is like. I've had many workdays as an RN in which I've spent more time doing "CNA" work than RN work. That's sometimes how it is. Yes, it's hard and it's humbling. Working at that nursing home laid the foundation for me. I wanted to prevent people from having to live their lives from a bed. I wanted to promote health and wellness. This, coupled with the demanding physical labor and low earning potential of aide work helped get me through nursing school. I am grateful as well for the lovely patients I met at the nursing home.

Chapter 5: Starting Out as an RN

Pay. When you finally do get your degree, pass the NCLEX, and start working as an RN, you will be astonished at the number of people who think you make tons of money. Shortly after I started working, I ran into a former neighbor in the grocery store parking lot who stated, "I'm surprised you're not driving a brand new car with all that money you make as an RN!" Also, because I work a lot of Sundays, fellow churchgoers hint to my husband that I make a lot of money because I appear to always be working. "Your wife must be raking in the money!" My husband also says that his co-workers think we're very wealthy because I'm a nurse. I've had patients tell me, "You must make what, $30 an hour?" Ha! You get the picture. I'm just telling you to be prepared for this. Also be prepared to laugh.

When I was hired to work my first nursing job out of school, I started out making $20.10 an hour. This was for a full-time, day shift position at a hospital. Remember, that's also with a BSN and no RN experience (i.e., my first "real" nursing job right out of school). A few months after I was hired, we all got raises. So now, just over a year later, I make $21.39 an hour. Now, if I do hit that over 40-hours in a week mark, I'm making $32.09 an hour. Not too shabby. But, recall what I said earlier about not killing yourself with overtime hours. It's really not worth your health. And your life. Or someone else's life because you're so exhausted you make a fatal medication administration error. It happens.

Yes, you can make some good money as an RN. Where you work makes a difference. Nurses in California make more than those in the southeastern states. Who you work for makes a difference. I work for a non-profit organization. Experience also matters. Usually if you've been a nurse a little longer, you can specialize or work for certain companies that pay more. There's nurses I work with that make $40/hour as their normal rate. So, don't expect to make a ton right out of school. Yes, you'll make more than a CNA, but not as much as you might expect. And, generally speaking, the higher your education, the more your earning potential.

Med-Surge. I started working my first job as an RN in June 2013. I'm writing this section in May 2014, so yes, I have survived nearly a year as an RN in the hospital. I started out on a telemetry (tele) floor and am still there. What is tele, you may be asking yourself. I tell people that I take care of patients who come in with chest pain and who have problems with weird or abnormal heart beats (arrhythmias) and I take care of people who have heart attacks or congestive heart failure flare-ups. That's mainly what we specialize in on 3 South. Buuuutttt, as a new nurse you quickly learn that everyone's got hypertension, diabetes, some degree of kidney failure, and COPD. It's just kind of how it works.

A tele floor is also sometimes called a "med-surge" (medical-surgical) or medical floor. They are similar, but tele has an emphasis on heart monitors. Most patients on a tele floor have six little stickers on their chest that connect to a little "tele box," which transmits their heart rhythm and heart rate to a remote screen in another room (the tele room). Yes, there is a person whose job it is to watch those rhythms for 12 hours a day and notify the nurse if something looks fishy. To be a nurse on a tele floor, you need to have some basic knowledge of how to read rhythms or strips in order to identify abnormal and potentially lethal heart rhythms. It also helps to have some knowledge of what medications treat what heart rhythms.

Three South is a cool place to start because it encompasses a little bit of everything. Every now and then, we'll see some really cool stuff totally unrelated to chest pain. One time there was a guy in there being treated for a snake bite. I took care of a young guy that got his arm caught on fire and needed antibiotics and wound care. And there always seems to be at least one person in there for alcohol withdrawal. Additionally, we see cancer, diabetic ketoacidosis, altered mental status, seizures, and almost any other thing you can imagine. I think one reason we get all those other-than-tele issues as the main diagnosis is because all the other units in the hospital are full. At least that's my guess??? And then, I've also learned that the heart is affected by a lot of things. That may seem obvious to some, but I guess I'd never really thought about it. For example, I took care of a young girl who came up from the ICU with the chief complaint/admitting diagnosis of "attempted suicide by drug overdose." The girl had taken a concoction of Benadryl and some other household meds and tried to kill herself. When people overdose, especially when they take things like cocaine, it affects their heart. One of my patients recently tried to kill himself by snorting tons of cocaine. His chief complaint when he came to the ED was "chest pain." The hospitalist admitted him to 3 South, put him on a heparin drip, and watched his troponins. All because of cocaine, they wanted to make sure he didn't have a heart attack. Cocaine constricts the coronary arteries and can cause chest pain. I don't remember reading about that in my med-surge class. Again, one more reason students should be in the hospital.

Nursing Specialties. I remember in nursing school that it seemed like a lot of my peers somehow magically knew from the get-go what area of nursing they wanted to go in to. I knew that since I was a little kid, I liked sports and thus I enjoyed learning about sore muscles, broken bones and sprains, etc. So, I thought orthopedics would be cool. During my second year of nursing school, I did a rotation on an orthopedic/post-op floor. It seemed to me like pain management was really the nurse's focus on that unit. And now I know for a fact (because I have worked briefly on a post-op floor when they were short-handed) that I could not permanently work there. It's all just about handing out pain medicine for 12 hours. And I'm not knocking the patients. But just be mindful that being an orthopedic surgeon and being an RN that works on an ortho floor are two entirely different occupations. I've seen some orthopedic surgeries. Super cool. I got to see a knee replacement and part of a hip replacement. It's pretty intense. Orthopedic surgeons are very very very specialized. As a matter of fact, I wanted to be one at one point in my life. In the OR, the surgeon operates. He cuts, saws, drills, bolts down, etc. He doesn't have to clean up the room when he's done or prep it beforehand. He doesn't have to clean his instruments. He doesn't have to prep the patient. He doesn't have to sedate the patient. The OR nurse, surgical tech, nurse anesthetist, etc. do all that. The surgeon just does surgery. The salary is not bad either, but I'm fully confident that they earn every.single.penny.

Anyhow, from a nursing perspective, just from that rotation, I sort of learned that I wasn't really crazy about becoming "an ortho nurse." And I tucked med school away in the back of my mind, since it takes forever to get through it. I could not work on a post-op/surgical floor. One of the things that stresses me out on 3 South is having to deliver pain meds to four of your five patients first thing in the morning on top of the 10 million other things you have to do. Not to mention that ever-nagging pain reassessment due within 60 minutes of the time you intervened for the pain. And then some patients have pain that just doesn't go away. Everyone responds differently to pain and it truly is subjective. But you will get those patients who watch the clock and don't really seem like they're in pain but you still have to take their word for it because you know that pain is what the patient says it is (according to a textbook from school). And for those who really are in pain, you feel bad when you've tried everything and gone to all lengths to alleviate it and nothing works. I almost get frazzled just thinking about all the call bells going off and hearing the secretary say, "Your patient in Room such and such wants something for pain" and then just running around like a puppet. Pain is a very interesting thing to research, though. I didn't mean to go on a tangent there, but I just say all that to say that as a student, you should really have an open mind going in to each rotation because what you think might be really cool and fun can turn out to be a nightmare. And even though most of your rotations don't last very long, you can still learn a lot. Try to see as much as possible and to really get an idea of what it would be like to work on that unit or in that specialty for 40 hours a week. You just might change your mind about what you thought you'd like.

Even looking back now, the worst clinical experience of my life was indeed on a cardiac floor during the second year of nursing school (semester #4). I had the most awful clinical instructor who existed to make me feel worthless (and she was good at it). I remember her going over telemetry strips and just thinking that it would take me a long time to understand what "a fib" and "sinus rhythm" and "PR-interval" really meant. I remember a nurse writing down on a sheet of paper what "CHF" was and the meds that were used to treat it. Wow, that was two years ago and I feel like I now know eons more now than I knew then (and I know I've only scratched the surface). That was the worst clinical ever, but now I'm working on a tele floor as my first nursing job.

And then I had some peers in nursing school that said, "I wanna be a pediatric trauma nurse and save babies on the brink of death." Sure, it sounds cool, but have you ever done that or ever been in that environment? Or some would say, "I wanna work in the ICU" or "I wanna help deliver babies." I thought my Critical Care rotation was among the most boring, at least for the portion that I was in the Intensive Care Unit. The nurse I shadowed had two comatose patients and all she did for 12 hours was check their blood pressures and then titrate their medicine on the pump. It was a lot of sitting. Probably the most exciting thing about being in the ICU was the bagels and the cream cheese that someone brought in to share with all the nurses (and student nurses).

Nursing is such a broad field. Maybe you already have an idea of where you'd like to work. I took the job on a tele floor because I had precepted there my senior year in school and it was in the hospital I wanted to work at and it was the only interview I got. But I can honestly say, and a lot of other nurses would agree, that starting on a med-surge floor is a good thing. You see a lot of stuff and you get familiar with and possibly even good at the basics—starting IVs, inserting Foleys, understanding common diseases and their associated meds, and other vital things like time management, prioritization, and how to talk to doctors. You learn protocols and start to memorize them so that what would freak most people out becomes normal for you. You learn how to do blood transfusions; you learn about electrolyte balance and IV fluids. You understand the basic stuff. With up to six and maybe even seven patients (on a really bad day), you have no other choice but to focus on what's important. When you're used to working on a crazy floor, like a tele floor, when you do eventually transfer to the ICU or somewhere else, it feels like a walk in the park. I've floated maybe three times to the ICU at my hospital when they were short-handed. I actually volunteered to be pulled one day because I knew it would be a break from 3 South. And I'm glad I did. I got two patients as opposed to the average five. It was indeed a break. My advice: Be a sponge wherever you start out. And don't be upset if you don't get your dream job or preferred specialty right off the bat. Start with whatever is offered to you and believe me, doors will open. It's nursing and it's a great big world.

Side note: It took me a long time to get this---the "floor" is a term used in hospitals to describe telemetry wards or medical or medical/surgical wards. It is different from the intensive care unit. When you hear someone say in the hospital "This patient needs to go to the unit" they mean that patient needs to be transferred to the

ICU. When you hear "unit," think ICU, where there's a smaller patient to nurse ratio. When you hear "floor," think of a big nursing floor, where patients aren't as sick and there's a higher patient to nurse ratio.

Orientation. Where do I begin in telling stories about my first year of nursing? I saw so much and I learned a lot. When I was first hired, I went through an orientation process, just like you would for any job. I had to give them my bank info and all of that kind of stuff. I had to get drug screened and all. We had to do computer training to learn the basics about how to use the EMR. New hires also attended a three-day orientation where we learned about the employer's mission and organizational policies and such. They fed us lunch too, which was very nice (cookies were included ☺).

In the middle of June, I started my real orientation on the unit. The manager had given me a packet of things I had to get checked off on week by week. I was originally told I'd work with one nurse preceptor for the whole orientation process, but I ended up working with about six different ones. They all had different styles, which is why I think it's good to work with so many different nurses during the orientation process. Towards the end; however, I worked mainly with Jo and Olivia, whom I liked. My orientation process was 12 weeks long. My manager, Sandy, had said I could make it a week or two shorter if I wanted since I had worked on that floor while in school and I was somewhat familiar with the flow of things. I chose to go through the whole 12 weeks, just because it's really nice to have someone holding your hand for a while when you're first starting out. There was soooo much stuff on that orientation checklist---code blues, code purples, code carts, blood transfusions, medication administration, making phone calls to pharmacy, getting report and giving report, assessment, charting properly, talking to doctors, talking to patients, talking to family members, locating things on the floor, etc. It can all feel a little bit overwhelming at first, but a lot of information is covered in that 12 weeks. It was neat to see how quickly it all came together for me, though, because I was actually doing those tasks by myself and they mattered to me. I also had a little peace of mind knowing that if I screwed up or missed something, my preceptor would come behind me and clean it up. Every couple of weeks or so throughout orientation, another patient was added to my assignment. New nurses on orientation start out with one or two patients and then are ultimately supposed to handle five or six patients on their own. It takes a while to get accustomed to things. I tried different ways of organizing my day and spent some time trying to figure out which method worked best for me.

The absolute hardest part of being a new nurse is that period of time just coming off orientation. It was very difficult for me. I hadn't yet discovered my routine, was still trying to figure out where everything was and how to get things done, and was still learning how to cope in this great big new world. Fortunately, I had some very supportive co-workers during the day shift.

Change-of-shift was the problem. I remember having to give change-of-shift report to a veteran night-shifter. It was awful. There was one in particular. I remember it was shortly after I'd come off orientation. I'd had an absolutely horrendous day, one of those days that make you want to quit your job. I think I'd had five patients all day, and they were heavy. My one patient was an African American man who had at some point sustained a traumatic brain injury and he was completely paralyzed, as you can imagine, and required total care. He was incontinent, had numerous pressure ulcers, was on numerous intravenous antibiotics, was in an isolation room, the whole nine yards. [Isolation rooms are a pain because every time you go into the room, you have to put on a special yellow gown and gloves, and sometimes also a hairnet and shoe covers and a mask. Oh, and of course you have to foam and/or wash your hands upon entering and leaving the room]. I remember doing the wound care for the patient, which took about an hour. As I finished up he said he needed to have a bowel movement. My heart sank because I knew that meant I would have to redo several of the dressings I had just spent so much time working on. That meant I'd have to take all my gear off, run to the other side of the floor to hunt down wound care supplies we probably didn't have, come back, gear back up, clean up the poop, and then redo all the wound care. And who knew, he might have to poop again after I finish for the second time, thus repeating the cycle. See how some wounds never heal? Anyhow, he had a sad story.

Another patient I had that day was an older white man. He had multiple skin tears that needed wound care that day as well. We'd also had a code blue that day on the floor that I got to help out with briefly. That patient went to ICU and eventually died that day. She was only in her 30s; I believe the story was that she had cerebral palsy. Helping with that code consumed some time, just as a code always does. In the afternoon, I got a patient from the ICU, a young black girl of about 19-years-old. Anyhow, I remember running around doing a million things and then having to deal with her blood sugar being really low. I was doing a lot of things to make her comfortable. I remember seeing in her chart something about non-compliance with the treatment of her type I diabetes. "Non-compliance" is a term we use to indicate that a patient is not doing what he or she is supposed to be doing for their certain medical condition, like not taking their medicine or using IV drugs despite a previous overdose. It's common. It's a nicer way of saying the patient is not doing what the doctor or nurse tells them to do (because it's good for their health).

It was a hectic day. The secretary informed me that the 19-year-old patient's mother had called asking to speak to her daughter's nurse because she felt like her daughter wasn't getting good care. I wanted to snap. Yeah, it was my fault that she was in the hospital. Uuuurrrr. Anyhow, I think I had a few other incontinent patients on top of all that. I ran around all day like a headless chicken. Twelve hours of it.

When shift-change came, I had hardly charted anything. I remember that one nurse grilling me about something stupid. I thought I was going to lose it. She was asking me why I hadn't done this thing or that thing and how come I didn't know what the patient's telemetry box number was. I thought it was criminal that any veteran nurse would treat a brand new nurse with such cruelty. There were a couple of them like that, though. Some wouldn't let you go if there was a little bit of urine in a Foley bag or if you hadn't administered the 1900 dose of sub-q heparin because you were busy doing something more important.

You've probably heard the famous saying "Nurses eat their young." This is true to an extent. During my time on orientation and especially coming off, I found a lot of the veteran nurses to be, simply put, mean. This was most widely observed during shift change, like I just described. I think the reason behind this is the fact that there's a baby nurse (like me) just starting out who knows nothing crossing paths with a nurse that's a pro and been practicing nursing for 30 years. They often have high expectations. They know how to get things done. They know what's acceptable to leave for the next shift and what's not. It takes some time to learn this. I don't know that they intend to be mean (maybe some do), but I think they see things and understand things differently than the new nurse does. You almost have to experience this to understand. I didn't even see it at first. Looking back now, I do.

I also ran into some veteran nurses who did enjoy teaching and warmly welcomed baby nurses. They make the world of nursing better. Mentorship is really important in this line of work. It's hard enough just trying to do your job. But to cross paths with a night-shift co-worker who chews you out and points out all your flaws in front of the patient really doesn't help matters (insert Taylor Swift's "Mean" song here). I've discovered that an older nurse who pulls me aside and lovingly teaches or gives feedback/correction is a real treasure. Hang in there if you encounter a malicious older nurse. Try to still learn from her without becoming a floor mat. If nothing else, my run-ins with mean nurses helped me grow a backbone quite quickly. I also used those encounters as opportunities to water that healthy no-care attitude.

Anyhow, that one horrendous day, I had to stay back and chart. I was stuck charting my 0800 assessments at 2000 (8:00) at night because it was the first chance I'd had all day to do it. I finally clocked out around 8:55 pm after clocking in at 6:52 am (a total of 14 hours 3 minutes on the clock). I was so ready to leave. Somehow I changed clothes so fast before leaving that I forgot/misplaced one of my favorite fleece jackets. I didn't care. I just wanted to leave. I finally waddled out to my car and made it there, in the dark, around 9:05 pm. I noticed a small note on my windshield as I got up close. I opened it up, as it had been folded underneath the windshield wiper. It was handwritten and said, "Learn how to park, Jackass, so other people can park beside you." The day wouldn't have been complete without that note. It was the cherry on top. My tire was just a hair over the white line that outlined the parking space. I drove home in a state of frustration, despair, and exhaustion. I questioned why I was in this line of work. People disgusted me. I wanted to just go home and crawl under the covers, locked away from the world of nursing forever.

When I finally got home, my sweet husband met me at the top of the stairs in our duplex. He had playing in the background

"Remember When" by Alan Jackson, one of the hallmark songs of our first year of marriage. He had the table set for a nice dinner. It had probably been set for hours. He'd probably been waiting, so lonely and patiently, for me to come home. I greeted him and through my self-pity and despite my disastrous day, I managed to squeeze out a fraction of what looked like a smile. I put my stuff down, kicked off my shoes, and walked into the bedroom. I couldn't help it. I let loose. The tears started flowing. I buried my face in my hands to try and hide the fact that I was crying. Richard followed me, like a devoted husband. He was hesitant, but asked if things were okay. Through my sobbing, I mumbled out, "It was a really bad day... A patient died." I told him about the details. Richard comforted me. I took a hot bath to unwind. He discussed with me something that would again replay in my head a number of times: "Babe, if you're gonna come home all beat up like this from work every night, you don't need to work there. It's not good for you and I don't like seeing you like this." My husband is my little prince. When I'm in pain, he's in pain. When I'm sad, he's sad. He's wonderful. I quickly learned the incredible value of having a solid support system as a new nurse. I desperately needed a companion that night, more than I ever needed one as a student. Anyhow, that day was very rough to say the least. I was completely spent physically, emotionally, intellectually, and spiritually. The worst part about it was that I knew I had to go back into work the next day.

While you're on orientation and even right out of it, try to figure out what your style is. By that I mean figure out how you like to organize your day. I know when I precepted with Kelly, she encouraged me to grab all of the medications (meds) for a patient and then go into the room and give the meds and assess the patient all at once and then chart the assessment in the room. Some other nurses I worked with seemed to pass their meds and then go back later in the morning and actually put a stethoscope to the patient.

One morning, I noticed a co-worker was done with her work early. I asked her what her secret was and how she organized her day. She said she went through first thing in the morning right after getting report and she'd go to each room, meet her patients, assess each one and figure out their needs, and then get into the rest of her work—meds, labs, charting, etc. I thought that was a good idea.

So, I implemented her system. I wanted to at least try it because whatever I had been doing didn't seem to be working too well. I started to work smarter. I'd try to get report pretty early and not waste a lot of time sitting at the computer that first hour of the shift researching every detail about each patient. Instead, I'd spend 7:30 – 8:00/8:15 going room-to-room and assessing each patient from head to toe. I considered that my first round. I'd ask each patient if he or she was in pain/needed anything so that I could bring it back for him or her with meds that I was going to pull. I started learning how to cluster my care and to make as few trips back and forth as necessary. On a large, busy floor (and 3 South is the biggest floor in the hospital) this makes a difference. Another benefit of this technique, assessing early in the shift, is that it gave me a good understanding of each patient's baseline early on. The floor is unpredictable; I could never tell when something was going to go south and the last thing I'd want is for a code at 8:30 in the morning to happen to one of my patients and then realize that that was the first time all morning I'd even been in the room (other than shift-change).

Know the baseline status of each of your patients—what

their rhythm is on telemetry, what their heart sounds like, what their mental status is, and what their chief complaint or reason for being in the hospital is. Focus on the big relevant facts, not all the minute, meaningless, unrelated details. This way, you'll be able to quickly recognize a change in a patient's condition and avoid sounding stupid when being drilled by a doctor during a code. It takes practice, but you'll get good at this.

Chapter 6: A Typical Day

My alarm clock goes off somewhere between 5:20 and 5:45, depending on how much prep for the day I've done the night before. I'm not rested because if it were up to me, I'd stay in the bed another 3 hours. I get up, though, without hitting the snooze button. I go to the bathroom, wash my face and brush my teeth. Then, it's back to the bedroom to get dressed in blue scrubs and compression stockings and socks. I put my badge on. Walk into the kitchen, get some coffee and water and start making eggs and oatmeal. Hopefully I made and packed my lunch the night before because I don't feel like doing it now. I sit down and eat a little something and read a Proverb or another section from the Bible. You have to feed yourself spiritually if you want to survive and thrive in this business. Around 6:20/6:25, I gather all my gear and head downstairs and out the door. I get to the work parking lot and park far away, around 6:40 am. I get up to the floor by 6:45ish and put all my stuff away—take my wedding ring off (to avoid getting unwanted contents in the diamond fixture) and put it in my purse and then put everything in my locker. I grab all of my necessary tools out of my locker: stethoscope and scope holder, pens, scissors, alcohol wipes, saline flushes, tape, clipboard. Then I go to the nutrition room the next door over and put my lunch up and grab a cup of ice water and write my name on it. I place it next to the sink along with my cup of coffee. I walk up to the front desk, grab my Vocera (our equivalent of the walkie-talkie). If I have an extra minute, I'll go ahead and print off a few extra of my cheat sheets. Then at 6:53 or so I walk to the Kronos, our time clock. I can't punch in until 6:53 am, but my watch is set a couple of minutes ahead. I wait then punch in.

    Whatever was before I came to work is about to disappear in the sea of craziness that is my nursing floor. I look at the assignment sheet with a mixture of anxiety and fear to see how many patients I'm going to have at the start of the shift, whether or not I'll have an aide, and how scattered I am on the floor. Then I'll usually sit down at a computer and pull my patients into my profile in the EMR. I look up a few things until the clock hits 7:00. At 7, I try to find the night-shift nurse who had my patients. I am a firm believer that shift-change should start at 0700 on the dot. At 7 pm, I'm ready to go, so I try to be courteous to the night-shifters and be ready to receive report at 7 am. Also, I don't like to start late. I jump right in and we go room to room and I get report on each patient. Right away, I can usually tell from that who my heavy patients will be.

After I get report, I go back to each room and officially introduce myself, tell the patients how to get a hold of me, and ask if they need anything at the moment. I also do my head-to-toe assessment then and see if anyone's in pain. After I've rounded on everyone, if someone does need a pain med, I'll usually grab that first. Then, usually by 0800, I start pulling meds from the Pyxis (the locked machine that stores most medications; all nurses authorized to use it have to type in a username and then place their fingerprint on a special pad in order to access the machine). And yes, I do often pull meds for two to three patients at a time (we're not supposed to), but I will not hold up the line if I know someone's behind me. There are three medication machines on my floor, all in different places. Often times, nurses have to run around to all three Pyxis machines to find all the meds needed for a patient. And sometimes the pharmacy is late bringing meds up, so I have to come back. I don't stall by looking up labs extensively unless it is a lab that's pertinent to a med I'm giving, like platelets for heparin or a Vancomycin therapeutic dose. And before I get too carried away, I do make sure patients aren't scheduled for tests that morning that might interfere with their medication schedule. For example, the night shift nurse should have told you in report if a patient is scheduled for a cardiac cath that morning. If that's the case, you want to be cautious about what meds you give that pt and you may want to check with the MD or cath lab first. Or if your patient is going to dialysis at noon, you don't want to give certain meds that are going to be filtered out (i.e., blood pressure meds). Usually, depending on what kind of day it is, I can be done with my med pass somewhere around 9:30 am.

    Once that's done, I'll usually grab a little snack and hit the bathroom. Then I'll try and knock out as much charting as I can.

Usually by 1100, there's another med pass. In between all this, you usually have phone calls coming from family members, the lab, x-ray, transport, etc. You have plenty of interruptions. Patients will need to go to the bathroom, you'll have to hunt down the kitchen staff for extra sugar packets, your aide will have forgotten to get vitals on a patient, etc. You might get an admission first thing in the morning, which is a mess, and in which case you might not get done with your med pass and morning charting until much later. I usually eat sometime between 12:30 and 1:30 and I try to make sure my meds are all caught up at that point.

After lunch, I'll usually have to pass more meds sometime between 2 and 3 PM. I am always checking up on my patients too, seeing if there's anything they need. I'm always trying to get a chance to read charts as well. I try to learn as much about my patients as possible. Patients get discharged in the late morning or early afternoon as well, which consists of more paperwork. Sometimes preparing a patient for discharge consists of hunting down the doctors if they forget to sign prescriptions. Pneumonia/flu shots are given at discharge time, and IVs and telemetry boxes get removed too. Either I or my aide (if I'm fortunate enough to have one) will help the patient get dressed. Reviewing paperwork at the time of discharge is important---it's YOUR responsibility as the RN to make sure that your patient understands when, where and with whom to follow-up and why; what new meds they need to start taking, and any other pertinent info. Then either I or my aide gives the patient a ride downstairs in a wheelchair.

Usually, if I discharge a patient from our busy floor, I know I'm going to get an admission from the ER shortly. So, I try to hurry back to my charting and make sure everything's good to go on that before that next patient does come. If an ER patient comes, I have to get the room ready, look up info on that patient, and get report on the phone. The patient usually comes at the most inconvenient time. Once the ER patient comes, it takes anywhere from an hour to an hour and a half to get him or her completely settled----tele box on, vital signs, admission assessment, admission paperwork (and most patients don't have a clue what medications they take at home), calling the doc, reviewing orders, getting the patient something to eat, giving the IV meds that the ER didn't give, etc. It's a process, which is why everyone dreads getting an admission. Anyhow, once that's done, it's typically somewhere around 5 or 6 pm. I then have to finish giving meds to all my other patients, including insulin with dinner. I make my last rounds about 6:15 or so to make sure the incontinent patients are dry and that everyone is settled. If I have to give a pain med to someone, I try to do that as close to shift change as possible. Aaaannnd if I have time, I try to be courteous and pass the meds due at 7 pm. I go back and make sure all my charting is good. By 7 pm, I'm back up at the front desk ready to give report for shift-change, which can be quite a chaotic time. It can take anywhere from 20 minutes to an hour and a half. Once it's finally over, I sign off on all my notes in the chart, head to the break room to empty my pockets and grab my things, leave the floor and badge out, then climb three sets of stairs to the first floor bathroom, change out of my scrubs, wash my hands, and head to the parking lot to hop in my truck for the 7-8 minute ride home.

Here's a peek at a Sunday 7am to 7pm shift that I worked. Oh man. It was a rough one. I started the shift with no aide. My patient in Room 3 was a 60-some year old man being treated for a pulmonary embolus (PE), and thus was on a heparin drip. His major thing was that he needed help using his urinal (he'd had a stroke in the past and had contractures in his hands). It seemed he needed to use the urinal a lot. My guy in Room 4 was very overweight. He was being treated for cellulitis an0d dehydration, among some other things. He was early-mid 60s, I believe. Room 4 (we often refer to patients by their room numbers) was a 90-something year old lady admitted for a CHF exacerbation/chest pain. Room 6 was an 86-year-old lady who came in for chest pain as well.

    So, the day starts out running around, getting vitals and blood sugars and doing assessments. The bulk of the morning consisted of running around helping people with toileting needs. Rm 3 needed help with the urinal, Rm 4 was incontinent and also constipated, Room 5 needed help getting to the bedside commode, and Room 6 very frequently needed to get on the bedpan to urinate. That was much of the morning. Oh yeah, let me say that we had 6 nurses total working. Two of those had been pulled from other units to work because we didn't have enough staff to start with. To add to that, Emily was made charge nurse. She'd barely been a nurse for a year and that was her first day ever being charge nurse. I was the most experienced one there of all the normal nurses for the floor, and I had only been a nurse 14 months. Fortunately, Pat, our clinical coordinator was in the tele room. I guess she had been called in too because she never works on Sundays.

At some point later in the morning, one of the pulled nurses got some patient from the ER who Pat said should have been a no-code but whose family wanted him to be a full code. That was a mess because it was clear if you saw the patient that he was on his way out. The family was a wreck too. I had heard Pat and the nurse caring for him talk about that patient's low blood pressure, which Pat said was considered a Rapid Response. Shortly thereafter, when I heard a "Rapid Response" over the intercom, I assumed it was for that patient, so I ran out of Room 6 after getting her on the bedpan and rushed down to Room 13 where that other patient was. All I saw was a room full of distraught family members, one of whom was wailing, and a patient who was obviously near the end. The RRT was not there. So, I ran around trying to figure out where it was. It was in Room 35, all the way on the opposite side of the floor.

When I got there, I encountered a patient who was passed out and not arouseable. The respiratory therapist showed up as well as the ICU nurse on the Code team. Emily and Rachelle, my two co-workers, were there too. Dr. Ewing and Dr. Ray were also present. It seemed the patient had been given too much pain medicine over the night shift. He wasn't responsive. He was suctioned and given three doses of Narcan, an opioid reversal drug. I acted as the runner, that person who asks what supplies is needed in the room and then goes and gets it. It takes time to find supplies on our floor. Pat told me how to get the intubation kit from the Pyxis, since I couldn't find it the first time. I also had to hunt down an O2 saturation device, since the one in the room didn't work. I grabbed a vital signs machine too.

The ICU nurse in the room asked me to page Anesthesia to the room and then to call down to the ICU and tell them we needed a bed for the patient because he was going to be transferred down there. When I called ICU, I told her what the one girl in the Rapid had told me. The nurse on the phone didn't seem to understand and/or was just giving me a hard time and said I had to go through the supervisor to get a patient transferred. When I told the one ICU nurse the response I got, she said, "What do you mean they're giving you a hard time?" The nurse on the phone said she would just come upstairs and see the patient because there was an issue with the beds down there. The ICU never wants to take patients. And then I ended up having to page Anesthesia twice. They never came to the floor, so the ICU nurse in the Rapid just said to tell them to meet us downstairs in the ICU. It was frustrating trying to go in between the nurse in the room and the nurse on the phone.

Anyhow, poor Emily. That whole scenario ended up consuming a lot of her time. When we were all in Room 35 handling that, there was a Code Green (which is a Medical Emergency) called on our unit at the same time. I was tempted to rush around and go to that, but I figured I'd better stay where I was at with the Rapid. I later learned that the Code Green had been called for a family member of the dying patient in Room 13. Apparently someone had become hysterical and needed some help. Hopefully that person was okay because most of us were tied up trying to help the patient who had OD'd (overdosed). Yeah, she was okay. Later, the OD patient was eventually intubated in the ICU.

At 3:30 pm, a CNA (and not the best one) came in. I also picked up a patient in Room 22 because Staffing decided that one of the pulled nurses should go back to her normal floor even though no one was sent in to replace her. The patient in Room 22 wasn't much of a handful, but nonetheless, he was one more patient, so I was up to five patients.

Around 4:30 pm, when I was sitting down trying to chart, the daughter of the patient in Room 6 came to the desk and said her mom wasn't feeling well. I went to the room (because it's what I'm supposed to do). The patient complained of a headache, which she'd had all day and just some general malaise (a general yucky feeling). We all believed it was from the Norvasc I had given her around 2 pm for her high blood pressure. The cardiologist had prescribed it. When I'd gone to give it, the daughter did tell me that her mom had reacted strangely to it before—that it caused her feet to get hot and tingly. I didn't think too much of it because it was a low dose. The patient later started complaining of chest "pressure". Sooo, I had to get an EKG because that's what we do. It showed normal sinus rhythm with a 1st degree bundle branch block...no change from her previous rhythm. I also paged the hospitalist, who told me to discontinue the Norvasc, even though the cardiologist had ordered it. I'd let them figure that out later. Then, the patient started throwing up. It looked brownish/red, a sign of blood. It was alarming. I gave Zofran, but the vomiting continued.

At the time all this was going on, it was around 5:00 and I was told by the secretary, so dispassionately, "You're getting an ER." Really?! I was in a sea of chaos trying to handle all this mess. An ER patient would make my 6th patient. I was overwhelmed. And I still needed to start my 5:00 med pass. I had to hold that one patient's meds because of the fact she was vomiting. The ER called while I was in Room 4 trying to hang his antibiotics and get him all situated. I was fumbling with the bottle and I had to mix up the antibiotic in order to get two grams into the saline bag. Pharmacy hadn't prepped it even though the nurse from the night before had asked them to. It would have made things easier for me. I asked the aide to change the guy in Room 4 because he'd had another bowel movement when I had just changed his whole bed at 3 pm because his sheets were soaked in urine and he'd had a bowel movement then too. I also told the aide that I was trying to prep Room 1 for the ER patient that was coming. She copped an attitude. When I ran up to the desk to get report from the ER nurse, she had already hung up. So, I called her back. When I got her on the phone and said I was calling to get report, the first thing she said was, "Did you read the SBAR?" She referenced some e-mail they had gotten down there that stated some new policy---that when the nurse on the floor was told she was getting a patient or when the ER called to say they were sending a patient, the receiving nurse had 15 minutes to read the SBAR and then to call back with any questions, otherwise the patient would just be sent up. WHAAATTT???!!! So, I explained to that nurse on the phone that the SBAR doesn't explain everything, like uh, whether or not the patient is alert/oriented, and whether or not he or she can talk or walk, along with other important assessment data and signs and symptoms. This is evidence of administrative people making rules without knowing how things really work because they're so far removed from the actual work. How is it improving patient safety to *not* give report? Anyhow, I had to deal with this nurse's attitude. I read through the chart some and then called her back in about 20 minutes with some questions.

When I got off the phone with her, I had to run around and try and finish my work before my sixth patient came up to the floor. Once that patient came up to the room, it was about 6:05 pm. At that time, I was back in Room 6 trying to assist my vomiting patient. My phone rang---a co-worker informing me of the patient's arrival. A second co-worker informed me of the patient's arrival. I replied, "I'll be there when I can." That patient's daughter asked me, "Are you guys short-handed today?" We're never supposed to say yes, but I was so obviously frazzled and overwhelmed that I said, "yes." Sometime during all the madness, my nurse aide had mentioned to me that the guy in Room 4 had messed the bed up in an incontinent episode. AaaAaAhHHhh!

Okay, when I finally got to my new ER patient in Room 1, I had to get her vital signs and put her heart monitor on and all that. Of course, the patient had chest pressure and was also starving. Once again, I was drowning in the sea of overwhelmingness. While I'm in there, I get a call saying that MRI is on the phone. I go to answer that, and the woman on the phone says the patient is supposed to go for an MRI. She had been called in to do it. I called the doc to see if that was an urgent test or if it could wait since

Transport was gone for the day. The doc told me it was an urgent test because he wanted to make sure the patient wasn't having a stroke. He wanted it done. So, since I had gotten no real report from the ER nurse and was rushed to read through the patient's info before she got to the floor, I didn't realize she even had an MRI ordered. Soooo, guess whose responsibility it was to transport this patient back downstairs where she just came from? Mine. Me, with five other patients---one on a heparin drip, one who was vomiting some sort-of blood-tinged stuff and also needed the bedpan frequently and another who was lying in his own foul excrement and needed total assistance. It was a mess. I had to hunt down some help. The patient had to go in the bed because I had to give her Ativan beforehand because she was afraid of the "tube" (i.e., the MRI machine). She needed to be sedated. So, I called the nursing supervisor to see if she could give me some help transporting the patient. I was really flustered, and mainly wanted her to come up to the floor to see how crazy it was.

All my co-workers were so busy and had heavy patient loads themselves. One of them was so kind and offered to help me take the patient downstairs. So, we had to take her all the way back downstairs where she had just come from. Urrr. We did that. I left the patient and went back upstairs because I was told the MRI would take 15 minutes. When I got back, it was around 6:45ish, I believe. I ran around and did a few more things. Shift-change report took a while. I had to talk to three different nurses. And, we had to verify heparin and go downstairs and get the patient from MRI and get her settled again. It was lengthy. My poor patient in Room 6 was still vomiting and apparently had been waiting on me for a while. She had to use the bedpan during shift change too. I finished everything up and finally clocked out at 8:10 pm, after a 13 hour 17 minute crazy day.

This chaotic day was just one of many. I believe it's a main reason that so many nurses burn out. Imagine this three (or four or five) days back-to-back-to-back. The most frustrating thing about it is feeling like people's lives are in your hands and you can't give them the help they need because you're constantly pulled in a thousand different directions. Not to mention the constant interruptions when trying to talk to a patient. What are you supposed to say when a patient's loved one sees you running around like a headless chicken and asks you, "Are you guys short staffed today?" It's never cool to make your employer/boss look bad. There's not really an easy solution. I think that's why so many jump ship. That's why I almost did.

I also want to take time to tell you about the conversation I had with my husband when I got home that night. First, I was hungry, so I stopped at Moe's on the way home and got myself two beef tacos. I got home and sat at the table to eat. Richard sat close to me, around the table in our dining room. I poured out my heart to him, like I usually do, but this time around it seemed a little different. We've had conversations before when I come home all frazzled and stressed out and I've basically dumped out on him everything I'd been holding back for the past 13 hours---all my frustrations, complaints, and annoyances. But this time, I seemed to step outside of myself as I explained all my issues to him.

I told Richard everything above that I just told you, about the craziness and disorganization of the day. I explained what frustrated me: It's difficult when you've gone to school for six years, spent $40,000 dollars for a bachelor's degree, studied your life away in a library while sacrificing time with friends/family, etc. so you could get good grades and be competent in your field, when you're young and energetic, passionate, and sympathetic, when you really care about people and want to see them get better, when you yearn to provide quality service and care, and all you see is people who want to die, don't want to improve their lives and get better, are content living in a hospital bed, are satisfied taking 20 pills a day for preventable diseases, and not participate in a relationship that you thought would work both ways.

Yes, I went into nursing to help people. But we did learn in school that there is such a thing as the nurse-patient relationship. I believe it is a professional relationship, but I also believe that human beings are intricate. We are capable of so much. I believe God desires us to be in good health (but I also believe that he uses sickness for His glory). We're supposed to fill the earth and subdue it. We're to be fruitful and multiply. We are to grow, create, thrive, explore, rest, dream, work, and learn. We are to live life. How can you do this to the fullest when you're ill? That's why I became a nurse—to help restore health and in some way, give people their lives back.

But what happens when you work with patients who are homeless and come to the hospital because they don't have access to medication? You see no effort in their lives to get a home, a job, or to offer a skill in exchange for pay. What happens when you discharge a patient only to see him return in a couple days? And this happens. All. The. Time. What happens when you repeatedly care for those who have been turned away by every other health care organization for dealing drugs within the facility and you have to care for that person for weeks because he has no other place to go? What happens when you repeatedly admit people who can't tell you what medications they take at home? And what about the uneducated ones that you're supposed to teach? What if they can't read? What if they have a 6th grade education? What about those who just got cardiac cathed for an MI but go home and still refuse to take their medicine, change their diet, and improve their own lives? What about the ones with no family members? And the patients with COPD, lung cancer, and tracheostomies who are oxygen-dependent who ask you to wheel them outside so they can smoke a cigarette? What about the "suicidal" patients that really aren't suicidal but just want someone to pay attention to them? And not only that, but in addition to all this, they are not paying for their own care. It comes at the expense of someone else. Where is the fairness? Also, these people express no desire to learn, to work, to live, to get better. It's often a one-way relationship. This is much of what I've witnessed.

And so, how do we fix this problem? How do we fix the brokenness of the human being—an entitlement mindset, laziness, poverty, homelessness, injustice, manipulation, etc.? I long to see people get better. Where is that desire in others? To live, to be all you can be, to experiment, to create, to procreate, to love, to run, to do whatever you want to do. Don't they want to live? I told Richard that I enjoy taking care of patients who are motivated. I love hearing, "What can I do to get out of here (the hospital) quicker so I can get home to my family or back to work, or back to playing golf? etc."

It seems a bit more rewarding to treat conditions that are not self-inflicted. After a while, your compassion tank starts to get low. You become jaded. You stop caring like you once did. I explained to Richard that I was not trying to complain or sound judgmental, but that I was frustrated because I saw no desire in people to improve their own lives or to lift a finger to help themselves. And it's very hard to help someone who doesn't want to help himself. To me, it's starting to seem like a waste of time. And talent. And money. And resources. What if we only helped those who want to be helped, those who would comply with the doctors' advice, instead of enabling people who have no desire to do anything but harm themselves? Is it offensive to expect others to take some sort of personal ownership of their lives and bodies?

Once again, these are things you're going to run into as a new nurse. Hopefully the people and situations you encounter will make you think. Maybe they'll make you want to change things. Perhaps you'll become involved in government because of them. Maybe they will make you want to educate people more and motivate you to teach a class somewhere. Maybe they will inspire you. Or maybe they will make you not want to deal with people at all.

Chapter 7: Shift Change

This is the time when a nurse comes in to relieve you of your patients. Remember, because nursing is a 24-hour business, someone must always be watching over the patients. Shift change is the time when you give a report or update to the nurse coming on to take over your patients.

I am a firm believer that shift change should start on time. Kelly taught me well and she was always ready to go at 7. I've grown quite a backbone over the past year and I no longer deal with a lot of nonsense when it comes to shift change. At 7 am, I try to find the nurse I'm getting report from to see if she's ready to go or if I can help her. If she needs a minute, I'll start my assessments or look up some more stuff on the computer. I have some nurses that aren't ready to do report until 7:20 or so. That's why I try to at least get a jump start on assessments or reading the chart so I know what's going on. The time between 7 am and 10 am is, I would say, the busiest time on the floor. It's not pleasant starting the day behind the schedule.

When I get report from another nurse, I use my cheat sheet and fill in what the night nurse tells me from her assessment. Likewise, I use info from my own assessment (documented on the cheat sheet) to report to the next nurse. I mainly want to know why the patient was admitted, what his mental status is, whether or not he is diabetic, what he runs on tele (the patient's heart rhythm—normal sinus, atrial fibrillation, sinus tach, etc.), whether or not he's continent, and what the plan is for the day. If the patient was admitted for new onset a-fib, I'm not going to hold up shift change because I need to know when the patient's last bowel movement was. Shift change should be short and to-the-point. Assessment data should be relevant to the patient's primary problem.

One night I went to give report to a float pool nurse. Typically, they have a couple years of experience in a few different areas of nursing. They're hired to basically go ("float") to whatever hospital or unit within the system is shorthanded or needs them most. They make about double what I make. Anyhow, I had been precepting a new nurse that day. I told her my thoughts on shift change and she seemed to be in agreement with me. This particular night, I think it was even a couple minutes after 7:00. We had given her report recently too. Anyhow, at the end of us giving her report, my orientee mentioned to her that she appeared frustrated or like she had whipped through report quickly. The orientee asked her what was wrong or if she was okay. That nurse replied, "No, you guys, especially YOU (looking at me), always make me feel rushed during shift change and I don't appreciate that, especially being a float pool nurse." My orientee replied, "I'm sorry we made you feel that way." I pretty much let her handle that and it's probably good that I did because I think I would have said something that would've hurt her feelings. The float pool nurse was kind about it. We finished report around 7:15 that night. When me and my orientee gathered our things in the break room to leave, I simply told her, "I. Don't. Care." I explained to her again that shift change starts at 7:00 and that if we would let that one nurse, she would sit at the computer for 30 minutes and write down every detail about every patient. I knew because I had given her report before.

I've had several nurses give me a hard time, saying that I rush them through report or that I "hound" them right at 7:00. I won't apologize for that. I'm doing my job. I am supposed to clock out by 7:30. And when I applied for my position, it said that I get off at 7:30. It says that night shift starts at 7 pm. So I have absolutely no problem starting report at 7. Any competent manager would back me up on this. It kills me when night shift nurses say they need to sit at the computer for "a minute" (which really means 15 or so) and look up information about their patients. No, they don't need to do that. If they do, they should come in early, but not waste my time. What if I had a kid in day care or an appointment or somewhere to be? They'd be costing me money by delaying shift change. They also cost our employer money because the longer they stall, the more I get paid (I'm paid by the hour; but really, I just want to go home).

By looking at any given patient's Medication Administration Record (MAR), it's clear that roughly 75-90% of the medications are passed during day shift. Day shift is when procedures and tests are scheduled, so it's when transport comes to get the patients. Day shift is when most family members come to visit, call and ask questions, etc. It's when doctors put most of the orders in. It's when patients are awake. It's when patients get discharged and the bulk of admissions come. It's when physical therapy, speech therapy, and everyone else is asking you how the patient is doing. Night shift is slower. Yeah, working at night is harder on your body, but the bulk of the work is done during the day, not at night, so I'm confident that the night shift nurses will have much more time at night than I ever will during the day to read the chart and research patient data. Besides, I give decent report and any important information will be relayed during that time. It's rude to hold up another nurse who has been working 12 hours, is probably exhausted, starving, dehydrated, and needs to go to the bathroom all because you need to look at the chart. Be confident in your fellow nurse that he or she will give you a good report.

One of the biggest myths you'll hear as a new nurse is, "Don't expect to get out on time." Yeah, there will be days as a new nurse that you have a hard time tying up your loose ends. But I firmly believe that if you plan your day and manage your time as best you can, you can clock out on time, even early. Don't misunderstand, things will happen at 6:55 pm that are out of your control. Your confused patient with a broken hip and with C-Diff will be up to go to the bathroom but will not make it in time. Her excrement will be smeared across the floor and plastered to the wall. You'll get called to that room 5 minutes before shift change when you had just rounded 15 minutes ago and the patient was fine. When you get to the room, the patient will be on the floor. You'll have to gather supplies, wait for some extra hands, gown up, and go in to clean things up. And chances are, you won't have an aide at that point and housekeeping will be on call. So, you'll have to make sure the patient's not hurt, get her up and off the floor, bathe and redress her, change the bed again, clean up the floor and the walls, take the trash out, get a set of vital signs, call the doctor, and then file that lovely little Quantros. Oh, and let me not forget to mention that while you're on your hands and knees scrubbing human urine and stool off the floor, your pocket full of pens and other supplies will pour out and into the mess you're cleaning up (yes, this really did happen to me). And then when you're done handling that at 7:25 pm, you'll still have not given report. Before you can find the next nurse coming on, you'll get a phone call from a disgruntled family member. You'll have to handle that and explain why you were too busy during the day to call her back.

When you finally get to hand-off report, sometimes you'll get one of those evil-nightshifters who want to nit-pick every little thing that they think you didn't do. Always do your best to leave your shift in good shape so that the nurse coming on after you doesn't have to walk into a mess. But at the same time, keep in mind that nursing is a 24-hour job. There are two shifts for a reason. I realized early on in this thing that I could stay till 10 pm or even midnight working and there'd still be more work to do. So be sincere in your work. Major on the majors---do what's most important and make sure it gets done, then focus on the little things. Prioritization is key.

Now I'll share a few tips for getting out on time: 1) Start your 5 pm med pass right at 5:00. And this means you can pass the meds that are due at any time between 4 pm and 6 pm, because we are allowed to give meds an hour before and/or after their exact due time. So, if you have Neurontin due at 4:30, Coreg due at 5:00, and Zosyn due at 6:00, instead of going into that room 3 different times, just go in once and give all three of the meds at once---5:00.

They're all still on time. Learning to cluster your care, as we call it, is an invaluable nursing skill. It will save you soooo much time and headache. Do as much as you can in the patient's room at once. Eliminate going back and forth as much as possible. I'm not saying to not round on your patients frequently, but do as much of your actual "meat" work as you can in one stop. Also, anticipate your patient's needs. If you know that Mr. Pancreatitis can have his Dilaudid again at 5:13 pm, take it with you when you go into his room right at 4:59 pm or 5:00 pm to do your last med pass for the day. By the time you pass his other meds, answer a few of his/his family member's questions, check his vitals in the computer, etc., it will be 5:13, so you'll be able to give the Dilaudid. Otherwise, you'll get in his room and have to run back out. And take another bag of normal saline too, because you'll probably have to hang it before shift change anyway.

2) That last med pass will probably take you 30 minutes to an hour. Once you're done with that, it'll likely be close to 5:30/6:00. Go ahead, and around 6 pm/am (depending on which shift you work), round on your patients, especially the ones that are confused and/or incontinent. This is the time that they like to go to

the bathroom and/or decide to climb out of bed. By 6:15/6:30, you should be good to go with meds; your confused patients should be safe with their bed alarms on and the bed in low position; and your incontinent patients should be clean and dry. Make sure everyone got dinner and is satisfied with it. Make sure no one who wants pain meds and can have them is without them, because if 7:00 comes and they're in pain, you'll have to run around and find pain medicine during shift change.

3) Make sure your charting is all caught up. This includes vital signs being in, assessments and pain reassessments being done, progress notes are done, and Quantroses are completed.

4) Remember, around 6:00 or so, you can peek at the assignment sheet for the next shift. Know who you're giving report to at 7. If you're on a big floor like mine, chances are you'll have 5 patients to give report on and three different nurses you have to give report to. If you have to give just 1 patient to one nurse, grab her before you grab the nurse who is getting three or four of your patients. Otherwise, the nurse you only have to talk to about one patient will get held up in report with another nurse who has to give her four really complicated patients and you'll be waiting

around from 7:20-7:40 yearning to talk to her for just three minutes so you can leave. Trust me. And don't forget, to save yourself a minute, type your change of shift note and pend it. You can go back in after you've given report and just sign it off.

5) Empty your pockets around 10 minutes before the shift ends. You'll be amazed at what you find. I've found little bottles of Ativan, heparin, insulin, and Dilaudid at the bottom of my pockets. I've found crumpled up papers of phone numbers of family members and lists of things I had to do during the day. Blunt tip needles (unused, of course), batteries, saline flushes, syringes, pens, markers, alcohol swabs, gauze pads, tape, Pyxis recipes of pulled meds, paperclips, and the occasional piece of chocolate or jolly rancher will all be found. You'll probably even find something you thought you had lost 12 hours ago. Return what needs to be returned and make sure everything gets back to where it belongs. If you need to waste a controlled substance, do that before the chaos of shift change ensues. I usually go ahead and hang my stethoscope and prepare my personal belongings for going home. It's the best time of the day. The main reason you want to empty your pockets before you leave the floor is because if

you don't, you will go home and realize that you've taken home a medication that the Pyxis machine shows you pulled and the computer says you never gave. That can turn into a revoked license. So, save yourself a nightmare and just get into the habit of emptying your pockets before you leave the unit.

6) Start shift change on time. Whatever time your shift is over, you should be ready to hand off your patients to the next nurse coming on to relieve you. Do bedside report. It's better for you and it's better for the patient. Shift change also seems to be when everyone has to go to the bathroom, confused patients decide to fall, family members come to visit, and codes and rapid responses happen. Bedside report allows the night shift nurse to say goodbye, knowing that she's leaving the patient stable and it allows the oncoming nurse to get a first glance at the patient and hold the last nurse accountable—that things aren't a wreck. And research has shown that bedside report is safer for patients.

Chapter 8: Charting

Also known as documentation. As much as I hate charting, I've also learned to love it. I remember being in nursing school for a short time and hearing the saying, "If you didn't chart it, you didn't do it." This is true. I found that documentation is protection from that evil night-shift nurse who wants to accuse me of not cleaning a patient or not giving a med or not calling a doctor about something. If it's in the chart, yes I did. On the same token, I don't chart things I haven't done (remember that whole principle of veracity that's a cornerstone of the nursing profession?). If I'm documenting in the MAR that I held (did not give) a medication and that I notified the doctor, but in reality, I only held the med and was planning to notify the doc but didn't do it yet, I DO NOT chart that I told the doc. …because I'm pretty sure something will happen in between the time I chart that and the time I thought I was gonna call the doc and next thing I know, I held some really important drug that the doc didn't know the patient never got because I really never did contact him. This can easily screw a lot of things up. It's better to actually do something first and then go back and chart it. Be cautious not to fall into "anticipatory charting" as I like to call it. This can get you in trouble really fast.

As much as possible, I chart in real time. This means I chart things right as I'm doing them. For example, if I'm in the patient's room at 7:34 am and I've just done my head-to-toe assessment, by all means, I'll chart that assessment at 7:34 am. If I paged the doctor at 6:15 pm to let him know that my patient had a six beat run of v-tach about five minutes ago, I open up the chart and make a note of that right then. Now, sometimes, as you can imagine, it can be very difficult to chart in real time. Like when a patient codes or an RRT is called. Fortunately, in a code situation, you'll likely have a co-worker who volunteers to chart everything in real time for you. And truthfully, I find it extremely difficult to chart my morning assessments in real time. One, because they're lengthy; two, because patients usually have to go to the bathroom or want to talk your ear off while you're trying to stand there and chart; and three, because you'll almost always be interrupted by something. So, what I usually do is open the chart and at least start charting my assessment in real time underneath the "Doc Flowsheets," which allows me to go back in later and know when I started it so I can finish it.

    Another great tool, in addition to charting in real time, is to always keep a sheet of paper and a pen or two in your pocket. If you can't get in front of a computer the moment that something eventful is happening, take two seconds and jot down on your paper when a patient starting throwing up or when the RRT was called, etc. And that sheet of paper will come in handy when a doc gives you a verbal stat order in the hallway. You can scribble it down and then get to a computer and put it in. That way you won't forget what the order is. I also use that little sheet of paper throughout the day to make little lists of things. If I'm in a patient's room and he needs 10 different things from me, I make a list so that I won't forget anything. Even make little notes to yourself that you need to go back and chart something in the electronic medical record. And keep track of the time. I try to put a time next to everything, even on my scrap sheet of paper. This way, when I do finally sit down to chart in the EMR, my note filed at 1800 can actually have little bullet points saying at what time intervals things occurred. For example: "1620 – Pt vomited large amount of green liquid. 1644 – Notified MD, got order for Zofran. 1700 – Zofran given. 1715 – Pt vomited again, small amount of green/yellow liquid." That sheet of paper will help you a lot.

If there's one thing that will make you late getting out of work, it's charting. So, one of the best bits of advice I can give you in this area is this: Chart every chance you get. If you've just helped a patient walk to the bathroom and she's going to be about five minutes, instead of leaving the room, you can stand there right outside the bathroom door where the computer is (a few feet away from her) and knock out some charting. Also, by doing this and staying in the patient's room, you'll make your supervisor/manager happy by preventing a patient fall and charting at the bedside. Chart any opportunity you get. If I'm sitting at the desk and on hold trying to get a doctor, I'll chart. And even on those crazy days, I will go into the Education Room (as we call it) during my lunch break and chart while I eat my lunch. I guess it still sort of counts as a lunch break, so you're a little less likely to be pulled away. I'd rather chart during lunch than leave late. Chart whenever you can. Don't delay because I can guarantee you that if you put off charting when you did have a chance to do it, something will pop up and the day will get crazy and you will wish later that you would have charted when things were "slow."

It's also a really good idea to document any time you talk to a doctor. If you notice a patient's potassium level is 2.5 and you paged the doc to get an order for replacement, make a note of it in the EMR. This shows that you were proactive and did what you were supposed to. Say an MD doesn't return your page after two hours and you call him again. Document that. If the MD calls you back but doesn't give orders, chart it. And there's a number of ways and places to chart.

Our hospital uses Connect Care by Epic as our EMR. It's user-friendly to me, and I don't consider myself super tech-savvy. Within the system is something called "Doc Flowsheets," which is where we chart a lot of things, like intake and output, our head-to-toe assessments, IVs, Foley catheters, tube feedings, blood transfusions, etc. The MAR portion is where we scan our medications. One of my favorite tabs is the "Notes" section, where everyone who works with the patient can go in and write a note. Once it's filed, it goes into the list of filed notes, in chronological order. It says who filed it and on what date and at what time.

The Doc Flowsheets is where I prefer to document important stuff, like when I called a doctor and if I had an issue with the pharmacy, if a patient was suddenly confused, etc. I've found too that the good doctors will actually read notes filed by the nurses. Sometimes physical therapists and other members of the team will read your notes too. It's good to document important things there because it allows other to know if something significant has happened with the patient. Often times, if I really want to get a point across, I'll file something in the Doc Flowsheets and also make a progress note under the "Notes" section about it too. Notes are easier for others to find. For example, I'll file a note and say "1410 – NG tube inserted at 60 cm. Pt tolerated procedure well." Later, I'll make an addendum to the note and say "1450 – Spoke to Katie, RN from Radiology. Placement of NG tube verified by X-Ray." There's also a way you can chart all this in Doc Flowsheets as well. It seems to me that fellow RNs that work the unit will often go to the Doc Flowsheets to find out details about an NG tube, an IV, or wound care, etc., such as when the tube or line was inserted and by whom and what a wound looks like (measurements, drainage, etc.) underneath the dressing.

To me, progress notes provide little chunks of important information in a more easily accessible place. It seems to me that the "Quality Control" people who make sure nurses are putting compression stockings on patients or are screening them for pneumonia during admission always check the Doc Flowsheets for that info. So, sometimes if you chart in the notes and not in the Doc Flowsheets, they won't see it. So, I guess it depends on who you're trying to please. Honestly, as long as it's somewhere in the medical chart, you've covered yourself. At least that's how I look at it. But check with your specific unit and hospital as to what exactly is expected of you. Just as there's an app for everything, there's a policy for everything. So it goes with charting. Know your unit's policy. Then if there's ever a question, you can say that you followed the policy. A great rule of thumb to go by when it comes to charting is this, which I was told in school by a not-too-shabby clinical instructor: "Chart so that you would be able to defend yourself in a court of law." It surprises me that no one really ever taught me much about charting. I think it's one of those parts of the job that's really important, but there's very little education on it. And that goes for the classroom, work orientation, and even on-the-job training. It's surprising. In school for a few clinicals, we would have to practice charting little notes on our patients and our instructors would scribble a few corrections on them. They'd briefly give us some tips on charting, but it was nothing real thorough.

Here's some more tips from what I've learned the first year when it comes to charting:

1) Be short and to the point. There's nothing worse than reading an ER nurse's note on every obscene thing the drunk patient said when in triage when all you needed to know was why the pt came in to start with.

2) Abbreviate as much as you can---and make sure you use correct medical abbreviations (sometimes I think doctors make things up). Oh, and I did learn in nursing school that "bf" is not an approved medical abbreviation for "breakfast."

3) Only chart what is important and relevant. If there's

nothing abnormal, don't sit there wasting time writing a story about the patient's morning. No one's interested in that. The only time I really pry open a Progress Note is like I said earlier---to notify a doctor about something or there is a significant change in the patient's status. However, some managers will want you to keep little progress tabs on the low maintenance patients even, just saying that you checked on them and that they were fine. Remember to keep your sentences short. Example:

- 0835 -	Called to pt's room; pt c/o CP as 10/10, described as "pressure" and "stabbing", radiating to back and down both arms. Pt sweating profusely and very anxious. 2L O2 applied, HOB fully elevated. BP: 165/92, HR: 110, O2 sats: 96% on 2L. EKG obtained, showed ST elevation.
~ 0840 –	RRT called. 1 SL nitro tab given.
~ 0845 –	Hospitalist called. BP: 160/90, HR: 108. Pt states CP reduced to 9/10. Another 1 nitro given.
~ 0850 –	CP rated as 7/10, pt less anxious. BP: 152/88, HR: 97
~ 0900 –	Dr. Strep present. Nitro drip and heparin drips started as ordered.
- 0920 –	Pt transferred to ICU accompanied by 3 nurses. Bedside and verbal report given to Dana, RN.

The above note says enough. It briefly states the problem and how I as the patient's primary nurse intervened to help the patient. It's not overly detailed, but it provides enough information to where another nurse who takes care of the patient the next day or that night would be able to get some good information. Keep in mind too that the cardiologist (Dr. Strep), who responded to the code will also file a note. So will the hospitalist. And their notes will be far more detailed and scientific than yours. In the note above, though, I covered my own tail so to speak. The note makes it obvious that there was a change in the patient's baseline condition and that I immediately did something about it (within the scope of my practice). I followed the correct protocol by calling a Rapid Response. I gave nitro, a PRN med, to relieve the patient's symptoms. I constantly assessed and reassessed the patient. I was proactive.

A few explanations of the above note: The "~" mark is what I use to abbreviate "approximately." "CP" means chest pain. Know that it can also mean Cerebral Palsy. That note is very similar to a real note I filed one day at work recently. Also, note that your employer/workplace will also have some way to report accidents or incidences. Our system is called Quantros. It's where we file bad things and even little details of what we're maybe not supposed to note in the EMR, like a patient fall. We also Quantros medication errors, when patients leave against medical advice, whenever there's a Code Blue, when doctors don't return your page, when an IV infiltrates, when there's been a HIPPA violation, when a patient dies, etc. You can file a Quantros anonymously and it's not intended to be punitive. It's really a way to track errors in the system. The higher-up people use that data to figure out ways of improving how we do things clinically. So don't be scared to file one. It will actually be used to help other nurses and patients down the road by improving processes in the workplace. And yes, I did file a Quantros on the above incident as well.

4) Don't make others look bad in your note. This means that you don't say what another nurse did or did not do. For example, if you page a doc and he doesn't call you back right away, don't chart, "The doctor didn't call me back." It's better to write in your note, "Paged MD to notify him of change in patient's status. Awaiting return call / awaiting orders." I was also taught that you don't want to chart what someone else did. Just chart what YOU did.

5) Please, please, please, please, proofread your note before

you post/accept/submit/finalize it in the chart. There's nothing worse than reading the note of a professional with the letters MD or RN or PA, etc. behind his or her name and picking apart the grammatical errors. Eeeww. Yes, I am a grammar junky. Proofread your note and make sure it makes sense to you at least before you publish it. Hopefully you won't pick up on any typos in this book.

6) Another great time that you want to chart is any time you give report to another nurse who will be taking over the care of your patient. This includes at shift change, when a patient is being transferred out of the hospital and to a nursing home/rehab facility, and any time you transfer your patient to another unit in the facility. Our EMR has built-in templates for this, where you just wrench in the standard note and then add in the nurse's name that you gave report to and signify where the patient is headed to. This is usually considered a "Routine Process" note. It just ensures in the chart that you didn't just leave your patient but that you made sure he or she was in good hands and under the care of another competent nurse before you left. Again, cover yourself.

There are also other situations where you don't have to record a note, but it's really not a bad idea. I always file a note whenever

I've received a new patient to the floor from the Emergency Room (an admission). My note will simply say something along the lines of: "1610 – Pt arrived to unit in stable condition, awake, A + O x 3. VSS. Denies pain. Tele applied. Pt oriented to room. Phone and call button within reach. Wife at bedside. Will continue to monitor." It's also not a bad idea to make a quick note for a patient who has just gotten back to the floor after a significant procedure, like a cardiac cath or even a thoracentesis (if not done at the bedside). Example: "1530 – Resumed care of pt after cardiac cath. Report received from Ally Small. Pt awake, A + O x 3. Dressing to R wrist cdi. Pulses present and palpable. Will continue to monitor." [Abbreviations: A+O = alert and oriented to person, place, and time. VSS = vital signs stable. R = right. cdi = clean, dry, intact].

Lastly, this might fall into the category of "anticipatory charting" but it is within the rulebook. Kelly taught me this as a way to get ahead in charting. If I have a few slow minutes an hour or hour-and-a-half before shift change, I will go ahead and pull up the template for the change-of-shift "routine process" note. I'll hit the arrows and type in the nurse's name that I'll be giving report to (if I already know it) and then punch in my name as the one who gave report and then select that shift change was given via SBAR report, ER update, Lab Results, Assessment findings, etc. Once I've keyed my pieces in to the templates, I'll hit the "Pend" button to put that note on hold. Once I go back in after I've really given shift-change report, I'll open up the note and hit "Sign" to publish it. It saves you a minute or so.

So, remember these things when it comes to charting: It's there to protect you. The EMR is a legal document, so take charting seriously. Documentation is your friend. Chart to prove you were taking care of the patient. Chart to show that you intervened when the patient was going south. Chart to tell a story. Be concise and to the point. Don't rat others out. Don't chart something you haven't done. Only chart what YOU did. State the facts. Proofread your documentation. Chart any and every chance you get.

One more thing on charting: A great tool in addition to your scrap piece of paper: your assessment sheet, one for each patient. Now, when I first started working, I'd scribble my change-of-shift info from the other nurse all on a little piece of paper. It was hard for me to read it if I had to look at it later and I couldn't pull out important data from it. It was a mess. Now, one good thing that came from one of those horrendous shift-change experiences with a more seasoned nurse: I took time on my day off to develop an assessment sheet for my patients. I thought about all of the questions she'd ask me during shift change that I didn't know the answer to. I thought about my own head-to-toe assessments and what info I thought was important to know for each body system based off of questions the nurse coming on would ask me. I also thought about things I wanted to know when getting report from another nurse on a patient I knew nothing about. I really wanted (and still do want) to be one of those nurses that gives a good report. By good, I mean, it had meat in it. You can leave the next nurse, who knows nothing about the patient, an accurate description of the patient. So, I have tweaked this form a number of times, but here is the one I currently use:

THE TRUTH ABOUT NURSING

Date: Allergies:

Pt: Age: M/F   MD/Hospitalist:
Code Status: Allergies:
Date Admitted:
Reason for Admission:
Hx:
Problem List & Txs

Labs:
    K+:   BUN: Troponins: WBC:
    Ca+:   Cr: ABT troughs: H/H:
    Na+:   PTT: Drug troughs: Platelets:
    Mag: INR:
Diabetic: Accucheck?:   Insulin scale?:
Blood Sugars:
V/S: Pain:
Mental Status: Diet:
EENT:
   -Glasses/Dentures:
Respiratory:
Cardiac/Tele: Peripheral Vascular:
   -Box #:   -Edema:
   -Rhythm: -Hep?:
   -HR: -Pulses:
   -BPs:
GI: Drains/Tubes: Output 7a-7p:
   -last BM: -Foley?:
   -bowel sounds: -NG?:
   -continent: -FMS?:
GU: -PEG?:
   -output:
   -continent: IV Access:
   -Foley?:   PICC?:

Skin: -blood return/flush:
   -wounds?:   -last dr change?:
   -dressings?:

Musculoskeletal: Activity Level?
  -weakness?:
  -deformities/fx?:

☐ AM Assess 12-   ☐ LDA   ☐ CP   ☐ PE   ☐ I&O   ☐ △

☐ D/C

Every nurse has his or her own little cheat sheet. On the floor we actually refer to them as our "brains." If you hear a nurse say, "I've lost my brain!", it means she's misplaced her notes. They give us the pertinent info. I keep one on each patient. It's a good thing to have handy during change-of-shift. You have all of the info you need. I always write at the top what the pt's room number is. I always want to know the patient's code status, age, when he/she came to the hospital and mainly why he or she came into the hospital in the first place (what symptoms was the patient having that brought him to the Emergency Room?). The table is something I usually go back and fill in later if/when I have time to read the primary doctor's note. I list what the patient's problem is and then what's being done to treat it. You can see all of the assessment data there. It's the meat. At the bottom, I gave myself some little check boxes so I can go back in and check off when

I've charted something, like my assessments every four hours. LDA is for Lines, Drains, and Airways (IVs, trachs, PEG tubes, Foleys, etc.). Once I check that box, I know I've charted on the patient's IV line or PEG tube, etc. CP and PE are for Care Plan and Patient Education. We are required to chart on these once a shift. My cheat sheet just helps to keep me organized and I'm familiar with this form. Create one that works for you. And again, I know some nurses who don't write much down at all. I'm not quite there yet. Also, I tend to remember things better if I write them down.

Chapter 9: 12-Hour Shift Survival Tips

A lot of the tips I shared on surviving nursing school also apply here. Of course, being an actual nurse is different from being a nursing student. For one thing, as a nurse, you're going to be on your feet a lot more. And for that, I recommend compression stockings. They are absolutely amazing. Compression stockings are made out of a material very similar to panty-hose (which I'm unfamiliar with). Anyhow, they're designed to fit tightly around your legs. Somehow, they keep blood flowing. They help prevent blood from pooling in your feet and calves, and thus they prevent spider veins. I've heard they can help prevent blood clots too. I'm not an expert on how they work, but I'll tell you I notice a difference from them. During my preceptorship in school, I didn't have them and by the time the day ended, my feet were killing me. They ached so badly. All I wanted to do was get off of them. My feet would ache so badly that I would start to get irritable from standing, the way I get irritable when I'm hungry. Anyhow, my advise: Get yourself a pair or two. Even try them out during clinical when you're in school. If you work as an aide or do anything where you're on your feet for a long time, they're not a bad idea. I notice a huge difference. Now I can't imagine not having them.

You can get compression stockings from medical supply stores, Amazon.com, and probably other places too that I'm not familiar with. You can get different lengths. I have the ones that go just up to the knee. Mine rest right below the patella, at the top of my tibia (again, know your anatomy ;)). Some compression stockings go all the way up to the hip. Try some out and see what you like best. I think I paid $18 or so for mine, but some are pretty expensive. I also bought a really cheap pair at one of the medical supply stores and they were noticeably cheaper in quality too. They kept falling down during the day and didn't provide as much pressure as I prefer. I think the ones I wear now are low-medium pressure. I do recommend buying some nice ones, though. They will make all the difference in the world for you.

2) Take time to go to the bathroom. This may sound obvious, but you'd be amazed at how many nurses go a 12 (or 13 or 14)-hour shift and only urinate once during that whole time. Nurses tend to be notorious for urinary tract infections. They don't drink enough water and they hold their urine forever. I myself have never had a UTI, but from taking care of people with them, they don't sound very pleasant. Remember, a UTI means antibiotics. Antibiotics mean diarrhea. And that can lead to skin excoriation. Diarrhea also means less of a social life. So just do yourself a favor and don't get one to start with. Practice what you preach when educating your patients, and take a trip to the bathroom as soon as you feel the urge to go. This works for pooping as well. Don't hold it if you have to go number two. I remember in Rehab class senior year in nursing school my instructor told us that nurses often have issues with bowel (and bladder) incontinence when they get older because of years of ignoring the urge to go.

An important tip on this for the real world: If you just "kinda" have to go to the bathroom or just feel a little bit like you could go, go right then. Don't wait. If you have the chance to go and you don't, I can guarantee you within the next minute or so, there will be a code or some other chaotic event that will take place and it will be another hour or two before you can go. So go when you can. Heck, even if you don't feel like you have to go but you have a spare moment, go anyway. Trust me.

3) Drink water throughout the day. Again, this goes with the last tip. As you know, flushing the kidneys out is good for your patients in preventing kidney and bladder infections. The same applies to nurses. Stay hydrated. And drinking water won't make you feel like crap. It'll make you feel good.

4) Sit down whenever possible. I've heard of studies that show workers who take small frequent breaks throughout the day are more productive than those who don't. So, I try to sit down whenever I can. It makes me a nicer nurse. Standing/being on your feet all day is hard. Managers and administrators who tell nurses they should never be seen sitting down are a little too far removed from the real-world of nursing. Yes, because of the nature of our work and the busyness of it, we do rarely sit down. Again, tired, achy feet are not fun. I am all about getting off of them when I can.

I've sat in the window sill of a patient's room while asking questions for the required admission database. I've pulled up a chair in order to start an IV. Now, I try to sit down when reviewing discharge papers with my patients. Another reason it's good to sit in a patient's room is that you can get on their level. It helps to show (at least in theory) that you're not in a rush. It shows you care. I've also, on a slower day, sat down in a nice chair in a patient's room and watched an afternoon TV show with him. We actually had a chance to talk about his military career too. I also shamelessly put my feet up sometimes while on lunch break. It helps reduce pain and swelling. When you do get back on your feet, you'll be glad for the little bit of relief you did get.

5) Chart whenever possible. I know I talked about this earlier in the section on charting. But it's important. This is usually what keeps new nurses from getting out on time. If you have a second, chart. Don't put if off.

6) Enjoy your days off. Rest. I'm not a huge advocate for working overtime in this job. The regular hours you work are hard enough. Take time to sharpen your saw. Sleep. Enjoy a hobby. Spend time with your family. Go outside. Cook. Whatever. Do

something other than nursing and enjoy having time off. Don't feel guilty that everyone else is at work.

Chapter 10: Miscellaneous Stories

I know I've shared a few stories with you, but I'll use this section as kind of a catch-all. I was thinking back on some particular patients and encounters and experiences I've had and what I should call this section. There's a number of things I could title it, like Screw-ups, Most Embarrassing Moments, Times I've Wanted to Quit, Difficult Patients, Difficult Families, Trying to do What's Right in Difficult Situations, Run-ins/Talks with Supervisors and Managers... So, here it is. You can read about my experiences.

PCA Pump Problem. One morning I got report on a patient

who I thought would be a fairly simple patient. She had end-stage ovarian cancer, had come from home into the hospital I think for nausea and vomiting (if I'm not mistaken, or it was for some other side effect of cancer treatment). The night shift nurse told me that she had spent all night trying to get the patient's patient-controlled analgesia (PCA) pump fixed. The patient had come from home and had been on an unbelievable amount of morphine via PCA pump there. She had her own pump from home but since she was in the hospital, she had to use our pumps. We on the tele floor don't see PCA pumps a whole lot.

At home, the patient had been getting something like 2 mg of hydromorphone (Dilaudid) every six minutes. To put this in to perspective, the normal dose of IV hydromorphone on the floor is 0.5-4 mg every four to six hours. Her daughter was in the room with her and was very pleasant. Unfortunately, the patient was still in pain despite being on our PCA pump and PRN morphine injections (IV). Pat, my clinical coordinator, knew about the situation. The issue was that the patient was getting so much morphine that our PCA pumps couldn't program to give that much. So, the pharmacy had to specially make the PCA syringes in a concentrated way so that the pump would take it. It was something like 2 mg of hydromorphone per 1 mL and the syringe was about 30 mL. The patient went through the syringes so fast, like within a couple of hours. I remember thinking, "Wow, this woman's already had 40 mg of hydromorphone since my shift started." Keep in mind that I'm used to giving hydromorphone 1-2 mg IV every 2-4 hours.

This woman was getting a TON of pain medicine. She was still hurting. Part of the problem, that I should have caught sooner, was that it took the pharmacy a little bit of time to create these syringes. I should have better anticipated when the night-shift syringe was going to run out so that I could have had the pharmacy working on it sooner instead of calling them once that syringe was done. The patient had to go I'd say at least 30 minutes without pain meds. That's a long time when your body is used to getting 10-15 mg of hydromorphone in that amount of time.

Once the vial finally came up to the floor, I had to figure out how to program the pump. The charge nurse that day, Amanda, helped me. The patient's daughter was getting upset because her mother was in pain and we were struggling to program the pump.

Again, the pump kept warning us that we were giving a massive amount of narcotics when the patient pushed the button and at a continuous rate.

Somehow, in the midst of this fiasco, Amanda and the patient's daughter got into it. The daughter and Amanda were comparing the pharmacy's label on the syringe to what the patient's order from home said. Amanda was trying to convince the daughter that her mother was actually getting more hydromorphone from us than she had been getting at home because our formula was more concentrated. The daughter was asking us to increase the amount the patient could get. Amanda explained that we as nurses cannot do that without a doctor's order. Attitudes came out on both sides. It was interesting that they went back and forth while I just tried to program the pump. Two nurses have to sign off on the PCA pump, they have to use a key to access it, and they have to use special tubing. It's a bit of work. Anyhow, we got that syringe going. Oh yeah, and the patient's sister was also in the room at that point. She was upset we had to wait a while to get the medicine to the floor, which I can understand. But, I learned from my own mistake there and called the pharmacy and asked them to go ahead and make multiple syringes for refill so they'd be ready when the current one finished, and so that the patient wouldn't have to wait around in severe pain.

The whole time, I tried to be polite. I was really just quiet. Later, I had to go back in the room just to reassess everything. The patient was still in pain. The daughter and sister were asking me how the patient could still be in pain. They kept saying "This is ridiculous." The daughter requested that Amanda not come into the room again because she was not pleased "with her attitude." I just kept trying to be courteous to the family. To me, it seemed they were more upset with the situation than they were mad at me.

Later in the day, the doctor showed up. I was in the room when he came. He explained that he would increase the amount of pain medicine the patient could get continuously and her PCA dose. He also explained to the family that the patient was getting more in the hospital than she was at home. I think Amanda was in the room too when this was going on. She and the daughter kept arguing. This doctor, one of my favorite hospitalists, was excellent in handling the tension. I just stayed quiet and listened. The doctor changed the order a couple of times to increase her morphine dosage. Eventually, the patient got up to something like 47 mg of hydromorphone an hour with her continuous rate and her own boluses. Unbelievable. My co-workers and I were so amazed that the patient was still up and moving and even breathing for that matter. And she was STILL in pain.

I remember the hospitalist (the patient's main doctor during her hospital stay) put orders in to do nursing checks every 15 minutes on the patient. The rest of us would be dead if we were getting that much morphine. One of my co-workers mentioned to me, I think it was Amanda, that the patient needed to go to the ICU if she was going to get that much hydromorphone because we did not have the man-power to reassess her every 15 minutes. She qualified for ICU. So, the hospitalist put orders in to transfer the patient to ICU.

When we got her all loaded up and in the wheelchair, she was in so much pain. I was trying to again adjust the pump to increase her dose. The pump wouldn't take it. The family was again frustrated because we appeared to be incompetent. Also, the daughter straight up told Amanda, "I don't want to talk to you again. I'm tired of you." Blaaahhh. I wheeled the patient down to

ICU with her family on board. On the way down there, I heard the sister talking about how bad we were at our jobs. The sister was already on the phone calling the ICU trying to get things changed. I remember giving report to the ICU nurse. The look on her face was unforgettable. I felt bad because it was like I was dumping a problem on her.

The patient hardly complained the whole time. It was the family. Maybe it was their way of advocating for her. I know they cared about her. Maybe they think we wouldn't have done anything for her if they hadn't been there. I can see their frustration. I was frustrated with the whole thing. I had three other patients who all had issues too. Oh, let me not forget to mention that my interim-manager, who was also the Director of Nursing, got involved. So did the Patient Satisfaction/Patient Advocate (Administrative) lady. It was a mess.

Remember, on a normal tele/med-surge floor, you'll deal with situations like this and have four to five other patients that you're responsible for at the same time. Oh, and don't forget that as a nurse, you'll want to make sure you've charted on this whole scenario. Again, you can start to see how nurses burn out.

I don't know what happened to that patient. And I don't really know what I'm supposed to say to somebody who's got stage 4 ovarian cancer, who's in chronic pain, and who has a poor prognosis. A few weeks after this incident, maybe it was a month later, I saw the patient's daughter coming off the elevator. So, I assumed she was still in the ICU.

Blood on the Floor. This next story falls into the category of screw-ups and embarrassments, but mostly screw-ups. I took care of a young patient (by young I mean like 30 something). He had some anemia and liver issues and a lot of other things going on. The doc ordered a blood transfusion for him. I got the blood from the lab and had my tubing and everything else ready to go. I remember I felt really rushed because I got the order for the blood early in the morning, during the busiest time of the shift. I was talking to the patient and went to spike the blood bag. When I spiked it, the sharp part of the tip of the tubing cut the inside of the bag. Sppllaaassshhhh. Blood on the floor. I tried taping the bag back together, which probably made me look more like a bafoon. I used my sound nursing judgment and concluded that an opening in the blood bag meant room for contamination. So, I ditched that bag; apologized to the patient; apologized, in my mind, to the blood donor of that unit; and called the blood bank back to request another unit. The woman on the phone would throw a hissy-fit, I thought. To my surprise, she politely said, "It happens." That made me feel better. What didn't was when she told me that unit was a special type of blood. Fortunately, it wasn't too difficult to get another unit. Sigh. The day carried on. The patient was cool about it. He didn't stress, yell at me, or anything. So, you, new nurse, learn from my mistake that you should be very careful when spiking blood bags. And if for some reason you lose your sterile field, start over. Patient safety trumps all.

Not too long after this incident, I came across this patient's obituary in the paper.

Chest Tubes. This interesting story is more like all the hardcore stuff that's shown on television. I had a patient who came up from the ER. He had a collapsed lung, also known as a pneumothorax. To get rid of all that extra air in his pleural space, the doctor had to come and insert a chest tube into that space. By draining the excess air, his lung could re-expand. I found out that the surgeon planned to do the procedure at the bedside, which I was totally unfamiliar with. I didn't even know they could do something like that on the floor. I was responsible for making sure the surgeon had all the supplies she needed, and apparently, I learned, there was a special kit that would be used for this procedure. Fortunately, the nursing supervisor was around for this, and she brought the supplies to the floor. The surgeon showed up. I'll call her Dr. Short. She's a general surgeon and excellent at her work, at least from what I've observed. She does appendectomies and other "general" procedures. She's very smart. I also love watching her interview and assess patients. She's very thorough yet to the point.

Dr. Short got to the patient's room and pulled up his x-ray picture on the computer. You could see his lung was collapsed. She talked to the patient about what she was going to do. He consented. We did a time-out to make sure we had the right person, the correct lung, etc. The instruments from the kit were spread across the sterile field on the tray. The scene took me back to my labor and delivery rotation when I was in school ---the delivery suite was set up with a table across from the laboring woman's bed. It terrified me --- a scalpel, scissors, that goose-neck instrument used for a pap smear. Eeeekk. It looked like pain. It looked like we were about to torture the poor guy. Dr. Short started by giving a shot of lidocaine under the skin to help numb the area. Think about any dental procedures you've had---sometimes numbing is the worst part. Not for this poor patient. He was only a little numb. Dr. Short proceeded by having the patient put an arm over his head. She then grabbed a small tube and very forcefully shoved it between this man ribs. The patient was not happy. He looked infuriated. For a second I thought he was going to punch Dr. Short. Once she got the tube in the right spot, you could hear the air come out of his lung. The patient finally got some relief. It was hard to watch.

When she was done and got the tube hooked up to suction, she left and headed to the nurses station to chart. I was left to clean up any mess she had made and any equipment she had used. When I looked into the patient's chart, I saw that he had no PRN pain medicine on board. I had mentioned this and the patient's wife seemed to freak out a little. "You get him some pain medicine right now!" Be prepared in this field to take the beating for doctors' mistakes. You will quickly learn that in this field, everything falls on the nurse. I mentioned it to Dr. Short who put some orders in. I was then able to give him something to relieve his pain. Relieving pain and suffering, is, after all, one of the main reasons I chose nursing. Do all you can to make your patients comfy. Any effort helps to build your relationship with them. And, I know I don't like being in pain.

Another story about chest tubes. I cared for a really sweet guy (in his 50s, I think). He had a chest tube I think for a pneumothorax. It had been in for some time and the doctor decided it was time for it to come out. The doctor never told me that he was going to remove it, but I had seen him on the floor and noticed he had been gathering some supplies. I had stopped by the patient's room at some point shortly after the pulmonologist (Dr. Raccoon) had been in there. "Aaahhh! I'm hurting," the patient told me. He was hunched over and face was grimacing. He had some not so nice things to say to me concerning Dr. Raccoon. "That fu*****g sh***y doctor is fu***ng killin me!" I told the patient I'd go grab him some pain medicine and be right back. When I returned, Dr. Raccoon was in there too. The patient wasn't happy. The doc explained that he was going to remove the tube. I told him I was there to give the patient some pain medicine.

Usually doctors will tell the nurse that they're going to do something for your patient so that you're aware and can get supplies, pain meds, etc. In this case, he hadn't told me ahead of time before he started manipulating the tube. Again, this is why it's important to round on your patients. I went ahead and gave 0.5 or 1 mg of Dilaudid or Morphine (can't remember which) IV. Dr. Raccoon continued a moment later. He was tugging on the patient's chest tube as the patient was yelling. "Are you trying to hurt me, man?!?" he said angrily. "Of course not," the doctor said. "It shouldn't be hurting you this much." After some wiggling and some pain on the patient's part, Dr. Raccoon had successfully removed the chest tube. As I watched the struggle, I really thought Dr. Raccoon was going to get punched in the face. The patient was in so much pain, even after the pain medicine had been delivered into his vein. Dr. Raccoon looked at the chest tube he had pulled out and said, "Oh, I see why it was hurting so bad." The end of the tube was coiled, instead of straight. It seems it had been scrapping the patient's lung tissue on the way out. Dr. Raccoon said he felt slightly embarrassed. He apologized, wrapped up the tube, and said he would show it to the cath lab people who had inserted it. "That's not supposed to happen," he said. The patient felt a lot better once the whole ordeal was over. He and the doctor made up.

I asked the doctor when he was done if he could teach me some things about the chest tube drainage system. He was happy to do so. "You want to see bubbling here," pointing to the water seal chamber. "You want to make sure this here is at 20 cm," again pointing to the water seal mark. "Of course, keep track of how much drainage you get." "And make sure you have no bubbling here," he said, pointing to the bottom chamber. If you see bubbles there, you've got a leak in your system and you need to trouble shoot. And if your tube comes out of the patient, you need to hold this petroleum gauze over the site and call the doc. Of course, you'll be able to tell if your patient is in distress and if you need to call a Rapid Response. And here (pointing to one of the chambers), well, I don't really know what it does. But those are just the most important things." It was soooo nice to hear a doctor say "I don't know." Ha, it made me feel better about myself.

An embarrassing story about a chest tube---I took care of a lady who had one. I was told by the night shift nurse that there had been no drainage overnight. We looked over the tube during shift change and all looked good. I got a call from the radiologist later that morning asking me to double check that the tube was still hooked up to suction because the lady's chest x-ray showed that her pneumothorax had actually gotten worse. I checked the tube again and it was good. The doctor told me they were going to have to take the patient and reposition the chest tube. I had Pat look at it. She discovered that the tube was clamped in one spot. One clamp was open and one higher up was closed. She had clamped the tube the day before. I was the one told to unclamp it. I hadn't completely unclamped it. Crap. Pat told me not to worry because her type of chest tube was different and that it was an easy mistake to make. She handled it with the radiologist. To my surprise, he wasn't mad. He said they were going to have to take the patient back anyway to reposition the tube. Moral of the story: Never clamp a chest tube (unless the doc tells you to ---and document it), make sure if it's supposed to be unclamped that it is completely unclamped, and learn from your mistakes. Learn when you screw up. It's okay to do it once, but don't keep doing it. I dodged a bullet on that one.

PainFULL Patients and Other Lessons in Customer

Service. If you spend any time around nurses while they're on the job, you'll likely hear them complain about "worrisome" patients. I hate to hear this label used because it is, in my mind, slightly disrespectful. Remember, you are in a customer service occupation. You're actually on the front lines. You make or break the patient's hospital stay. But, the point is, it's true. You will, just as in any job, have your share of difficult customers. Some of them are legitimately time-consuming because of important health issues, others have difficult family members that nag you all day long, others will ask you to do little tasks that are time-consuming but unimportant, etc. You get my point. Here's my experiences with "difficult" patients and how I served them.

Something you'll learn quickly on a med-surge floor is that some people are addicted to pain medicine. This to me, is one of the most difficult patients to care for. I don't mind caring for the 85-year-old lady who has bone cancer and needs her Oxycontin and morphine every few hours, but it's a different thing to have a 30-year-old who's addicted to Percocet because it's been abused. I took care of a guy who was in his 40s or 50s (I can't remember).

Anyhow, he was in rough shape. He told me his story…that he had sustained some injury while at his job. He also had neuropathy. Anyhow, he was on pain medicine at home. We were also giving him PO pain meds in the hospital. He was complaining that we weren't giving him enough. I reassured him that I would let the doctor know. I believe I ended up calling the doctor instead of waiting for him to come to the floor. This patient was nuts. You'll often hear of "clock-watchers." He was one. If I was not in his room the moment his pain med was due, he would start shouting my name out in the hallway. And he was heard by all. Keep in mind, I had three to four other patients. If you have a patient who CAN get pain meds every hour or two etc. and they know that, they will work it. I wondered if this guy was really in pain. Or maybe he was just bored. But no joke, it was every time. The very second his pain med was due, he would be on the call button and/or be calling my name out in the hallway. I had a talk with him. I think the doc did increase his dose by a little bit. When I was late giving his pain med, he snobbishly said, "Oh, you can give me another dose sooner now because you're late with this dose." Oh. My. Word. I had to explain to him that it didn't work that way. We ended up getting along okay.

If you're ever really frazzled because a patient is upset with you that they're not getting pain meds or enough pain medicine, just mention it to the doctor. Have the doctor explain to them WHY he will not increase the dose. A lot of times if they hear it from the doctor, it clears things up for you and you can become a little less of a scapegoat. "Seeee, it's true that I can't adjust your dose of pain medicine. The doctor does that. I'm not the one who's been withholding it. It's the doctor." Again, this isn't to point the finger. But seriously, hospitalists need to have a conversation with their pain patients as to why they can't have more morphine or Percocet. It will also keep you as the nurse from having to listen to the patient complain all shift and from having to call the doctor constantly to adjust the meds. Clear communication helps us all.

I had another similar patient. He was a young guy. His story was that he'd had some surgery on his leg (a while ago) and that he was always in pain. The IV pain medicine we were giving him wasn't enough. He was another guy that would call out if his nurse wasn't there on the dot---with Ativan and morphine. I had to explain to him that I could not just give him more pain medicine without an order. "Well, can you call the doctor right now and have him increase the pain medicine? I'm hurting." "Um, okay, I'll talk to him and see what we can do for ya, okay?" "So you're gonna go call him now, right?" "I have to round on some other patients and check on them first. But I'll work on it for ya." I was trying to buy myself some time. You have to read how urgent things are.

Doctors usually don't move faster for patients that are seeking pain meds. If it's a patient that has no PRN pain medicine on board and he or she has a headache or was diagnosed with a PE, they'll usually say right on the phone to give something or they'll put the order in for you right away. For more complex patients, they have to look at renal and liver function first and also assess the patient's history; sometimes they're already aware of the ones that just want pain meds. I did page the hospitalist. He said he'd come and see the patient.

Meanwhile the patient had called me back to his room. "So, the doctor's coming now to talk to me? Can I get some more Ativan and Morphine?" "It's not time yet; I just gave it less than an hour ago." "But did you tell the doctor I'm hurting?" On and on it went. This guy thought he was my only patient.

Eventually, the doctor came to see him. Everything I told the doc was confirmed in their interaction. I stood right there. The hospitalist explained that he was not going to increase the dose of IV pain medicine because he did not want to harm the patient and cause further addiction problems. He mentioned getting the patient referred to a pain clinic. The patient wasn't happy and asked for another doctor. Dr. Ho explained that he could request another doctor and that I could help the patient get a new hospitalist. Later, I did give the patient the phone number for Patient Services so that he could file a complaint. I stood with the doctor, though. He was skeptical and so was I. Anyhow, I still was left for another six hours with the patient while the doctor got to leave after spending about one or two minutes in there. Uhhhh.

At other times, I care for patients who just can't get comfortable. One lady I cared for recently had been in the hospital for months. She had chronic back pain. Repositioning didn't help much. She was another one that would call out "Nuuuurrrrrrsssseee!!!!" very often. Everyone would hear and I'd get about three phone calls, an overhead page, and about two or three co-workers, plus the patient's husband at the desk, all telling me to go to the room because she needed pain medicine. "I was just in there, and I can't give her pain meds again for another 30 minutes," I'd tell each one. My blood pressure would increase. "Nuuuurrrrsseeee!!!!!" The lady could get up to 4 mg of IV Dilaudid every hour. She was still hurting. I was using a heat pad too for her back. I suggested to the hospitalist that we use a PCA pump for her. "But then we won't be able to discharge her," I was told. Our hospital policy states that patients have to be off the PCA pump for 24 hours prior to discharge. A few days later, the patient went to the ICU. I don't really think she was on her way out of the hospital.

I recently took care of a difficult patient. She was in her 30s and had been admitted the night before for nausea, vomiting, abdominal pain, and diarrhea. Before I had even got report on her, though, my aide came to me and said she was requesting pain medicine. I found the night shift nurse a few rooms down and asked if I could pull pain medicine right quick. Before I could get to that, though, I was distracted by something else. Anyhow, I ended up getting report on this young gal. All seemed okay.

Doctors were thinking pancreatitis. The patient was on isolation to rule-out C-Diff, a really nasty form of diarrhea. The night shift nurse told me that she explained the contact precautions to the patient and that she was okay with it and understood everything.

After getting report, I introduced myself and told the patient that I would go grab her pain medicine and be back quickly. I also asked if she needed anything else. I came back shortly with Dilaudid, Zofran, and Protonix. I explained to her what each med was for. I assessed her and listened to her tell me about her admission. We got along well, like we were friendly neighbors exchanging conversation. I concluded our interaction by saying I'd be back in an hour to check on her.

When I peeked by to reassess her pain, she was asleep. A little later, transport came to take her downstairs for an abdominal ultrasound. When she got outside her room, she appeared perplexed by the isolation cart. I re-stated what the precautions were for. She was also aware of why she was having an abdominal ultrasound. So, she hopped on the stretcher and was wheeled down the hall by another staff member.

A little later, I was informed that the patient was back on

the floor. Within about 10 minutes, I went back into the room to check on her. It seemed that she had turned into someone else. "Man, my stomach hurts and y'all are doing anything about it. No one's telling me what's going on. I'm hungry. I'm uncomfortable! No doctor has been in here to talk to me. Y'all have just been giving me all this medicine and not telling me what it's for! I told the technician downstairs that he was hurting my stomach and he still went on with the test! "Um, ma'am, well, I haven't yet read through all of your chart…" "Man, what you mean, you been givin' me all these drugs and you don't even know what's going on with me! I wanna talk to the AOD (her term for Administrator on Duty; I think she meant Director of Nursing, the head honcho). I replied calmly and in a soft voice, "Well, let me re-phrase that. I haven't read all of the doctor's notes yet, but we are treating your symptoms and doing some tests in order to really figure out what's going on…" "Well, get my doctor up here to talk to me. I'm in pain and y'all aint doin anything about it." "Well, ma'am, remember earlier, I gave you some Dilau…" "You don't care about my pain! I wanna talk to your supervisor. Meanwhile, she proceeded to pull out her cell phone and call the Patient Advocacy office downstairs. She was so snappy. I told her I would work on some of these issues for her. It was nearly impossible to talk sensibly *with* her.

I called the PA who was seeing her and expressed that she had some questions for him and that she was in a lot of pain. He said he would be up shortly and see her first. Later, he told me that she was upset and that he reassured her that she did not have cancer. He told me she was better (emotionally) after he spoke to her. He also increased her pain medicine.

I went back in the room shortly thereafter. She was soooo upset. She commented that she was still uncomfortable. "Get me my pain medicine. The doctor just increased the dose. You still didn't get your supervisor in here!" "Well, the doctor just spoke to you, huh?" "You know what, I'm tired of your sarcasm! I don't wanna see you anymore." The "f" word was mixed in with her tirade. "I want a new nurse! I'm gonna check out of here." At some point in all of this, I heard her talking to the patient care rep on the phone, "I'm dissatisfied with the care I've been getting. I'd like to talk to somebody. Oh, so are all of y'all incompetent?" She switched back to me. I tried a little more to interject and explain some things. She didn't want to hear it. "Everyone else is right. This hospital does suck. The other hospital *is* better." Whenever patients say this I really have to practice some self-control when all the while in my mind I'm thinking, *Well, it's right down the street. Why don't you just wheel yourself on down there?* I guess I wouldn't have my job too long if I said what I thought, though. "I'm requesting a different nurse." I said in a perplexed/confused tone, "Okaaay, we can do that." I left the room without really even finishing the conversation. It was a waste of time trying to talk sensibly with this woman.

    I did the right thing and went to the charge nurse for the day and told her what was going on. I asked if I could switch patients with someone. She told me to talk it over with Pat, the clinical coordinator. I did. She tweaked the assignment so that me and a co-worker would switch patients. I explained the situation to both of them and that I really didn't get what I had done to cause the girl to snap. Pat asked me if she was bipolar. The girl had no psych history listed. Also, when Pat learned that the patient had pancreatitis, she thought some of her behavioral/emotional backlash toward me may have been related to possible alcohol withdrawal. But there was no ETOH (alcohol) history listed. But then I wonder if the girl maybe had been dishonest about drinking. Nearly every case of pancreatitis that I've seen in my short career was alcohol-induced. I had pulled more Dilaudid for the patient. I gave it to Pat and asked if she could go in there and give the medicine and talk to her for me. Pat's awesome. She did. She later told me that I had done something to upset the girl. She reported to Pat that I was sarcastic. Pat said, "I've never known you to be sarcastic." (I can be sarcastic at times, but it's usually quite obvious when I am and I do it in a joking manner, not in a mean way toward people).

In the case of this girl, I was just confused more than anything. Before she went to Ultrasound, she and I were alright. We were talking about school and God. We hit it off well. It was like she was a different person when she came back. Once she was removed from my assignment, I shook the thing off and carried on with my day. It still bothered me. Had I done something wrong? I was comforted, though, a few days later, when I heard some fellow nurses saying that she was a little bit needy or a little bit off. Later in the week, I was told that patient ended up leaving against medical advice (AMA).

My Advice. Sometimes it can be hard, but you have to take a patient's complaint of pain seriously. You will take care of people who are addicted to narcotics. They will nag you to death and expect you to be in the room on the dot with their pain meds. You'll wonder, as I have and still do what some patients do at home. How do they manage their pain? I've had some tell me that they just live with the pain (but I guess they expect a miracle cure in the hospital???). I am convinced that some of my patients, if they had access to IV pain meds and an endless supply of pain-relieving pills, that they would kill themselves trying to drown their pain. It's really quite sad.

Some patients don't understand that you cannot adjust medication dosages. Doctors do that. As the nurse, one of the best things you can do for a patient who is in pain is express that you care. State back to them where they've said their pain is, how bad it hurts on a scale of 1-10 (if the patient is verbal), as well as what their preferences are in terms of pain medication-type, amount, route, and frequency of the drug. Do this because you really do care and because it's important information. And don't forget that medicine is not the only thing that relieves pain. Ice is wonderful for sprains. Heat is great for tight muscles. Jerry-rig together an ice pack or a heat pad and bring it to your patient who is in pain. Dim the lights. Elevate a sore extremity. Reposition the patient. Throw an extra pillow in the bed. You'd be amazed at how some of the little, "less extreme" interventions help alleviate pain. Ha, I've noticed that distracting some people helps too. Start talking about sports or grandchildren or even the weather. If your patient has something to think about other than pain, suddenly he or she may hurt a little less.

Also, make sure that before you call the doctor requesting a pain med that there is nothing listed under PRN Meds. Also, check the doctor's latest progress note. Maybe there's a reason he or she is withholding pain medicine---poor kidney or liver function, past pain-med seeking behavior, allergies, etc. Investigate. Do this for your patient and for you---so you don't look like an idiot when you call the doctor and he has to say something that he's already documented.

In situations like the above, you'll want to snap on people. You will have days where you've done nothing wrong and patients are still mad at you. You will be pooped on (literally), thrown up on (literally), cursed at, berated, interrogated, and criticized. You will hear patients and their loved ones talk about you while you're in the room and talk about how lousy your organization is while you're in the room working and serving their loved one. You'll have people pester you at the front desk and make you look lazy in front of all your co-workers when you've been busting your butt and working hard all day. You're gonna feel like giving people a piece of your mind. You're gonna feel like telling them to go AMA, to check out on their own, to go to another hospital if ours is so bad. Fill in the blank.

Believe me when I say, it's always best to hold your tongue. I recently found a Bible verse that has helped me in this. I've written it down. I meditated on it the other day while on the job and it helped a lot. Ephesians 6:6-8 – "Don't work only while being watched, in order to please men, but as slaves of Christ, do God's will from your heart. Render service with a good attitude, as to the Lord and not to men, knowing that whatever good each one does, slave or free, he will receive this back from the Lord." The apostle Paul was instructing slaves here in this scripture, but I think it's a good verse for nurses to know too. Also, I think about when Jesus said, "Whatever you did to the least of these (the hungry, the thirsty, the naked, the alien, the inmate, the sick), you did unto me" (Matthew 25:34-40).

I'm serving Jesus. I need to look past the outward appearance. I haven't walked in this patient's shoes. No, I don't have cancer or renal failure or heart failure. No, I'm not bedridden. No, I'm not demented. No, I'm not 90 years old, addicted to drugs, oxygen-dependent, on welfare. And neither do I know what it's like to have a loved one in that place. Endure. Hold your tongue. Love people. It's easy when staffing is good, your patient loves you, and family members are sweet and helpful. But remember, this line of work will expose you to people in their worst states. They could be days from death or one more missed bill away from losing their house or one more sick day away from losing their job. You never know. But I can almost guarantee that whatever they have going on, it's probably a lot harder than whatever you're going through. So do the best you can for them. Remember why you chose nursing. Be the hands and feet of those who can't do for themselves. Be compassionate. Do it unto the Lord.

One more thing, on the note of customer service. I know how much it bothers me when I'm paying for something, whether it be food, a flight, a movie, etc., and the person serving me has a bad attitude. Uuuuhhhh. I always think, "I'm paying for this!" Vice versa. When I clock in everyday, I belong to my company. They are paying me to provide a service. My job responsibilities are clear. And yeah, there are plenty of days I feel overworked and underpaid. But, I'm being paid. Always try to imagine yourself on the other end. What if you were the one in the hospital bed? What if it were your mom in the hospital bed? Your grandfather? Your son? Your daughter? Your best friend? So, be that nurse with a good attitude. Be respectful. Talk nicely to people. Show you care.

Shaved Head. As you can imagine, nursing can be sad. And death is not the only reason why it is sad. I took care of an elderly lady who was on isolation for bed bugs and lice. The story I had heard was that her daughter had not been looking after her properly. The home the patient had been staying in had been infested with bugs. When it came time to discharge the patient, the case managers had arranged for her to go to a nursing home. I was told that before she could leave the hospital, she had to be completely cleared of having bed bugs. The doctor asked me to re-examine her scalp and skin. I remember running my fingers through her thin, short hair. There were scabs and scratches, evidence of itching. She had dead lice in her pubic area. The patient asked me to shave off all of her hair before she left. I borrowed an electric razor from the ICU.

I talked things over with the patient and made sure that she wanted me to shave her head. She was in her right mind, so I proceeded to shave her head. (I charted this in a progress note too). Her hair was already short but she wanted it all gone. I used the razor and completely shaved off her hair. She felt her head at the end and said that she was content with it. It made me so sad, though. Hair is a woman's pride, just like a mane is for a lion. Her head was completely bare. She was a frail woman who had not been properly cared for. It made me sad that we even had to talk about cutting her hair in the first place. She left us and went on to the nursing home.

Munchausen Syndrome. On and off for what seemed like a few weeks, I overheard my co-workers and even my manager complain about a patient on the floor. "Uhh, that lady wants her pain medicine again." I was a little curious. One day it was my turn to have this difficult patient. The night-shift nurse who gave me report on her said very clearly, "I am back tonight and I do not want her back on my assignment."

Anyhow, the lady was Caucasian, in her sixties, and had been admitted for nausea and abdominal pain. She'd been in the hospital for weeks and had appealed her discharge twice. Doctors had run every relevant test on her to address her concerns and to make sure nothing was wrong. Anyhow, we had treated her for a UTI (Urinary Tract Infection) during her stay but it was clear that she no longer needed to be in the hospital. I introduced myself to her and resumed care of her. She was very particular about her medications, saying that she had to take one before the other and then the next pill 30 minutes after eating. She refused to take the hospital's version of certain drugs. She needed pain medicine every few hours, but Dilaudid didn't seem to help her pain. She didn't want to eat. She refused to have an abdominal ultrasound done. She was paranoid about her UTI and thought that it was eating her internal organs. Doctors reassured her otherwise. She had asked multiple nurses to speak with the doctor about increasing her pain medicine. Doctors didn't want to for one reason or another. She continually asked me to call the doctor for more pain medicine. This has already been done by other nurses, though, and they were all aware of her situation. I brought her ice packs to try to express concern and told her that she needed to ask the doctor when he came in about pain medicine. I told her that the doctors did not want to give her more pain meds. Eventually, they took her off the Dilaudid and she was not happy about it.

Anyhow, it came time to discharge her for real. It was the third time that she had been discharged. The case manager told me that she had to go and that the transport company was being arranged for her. She was not happy about leaving and tried so hard to make the discharge process difficult. "Well, I take more Synthroid than this prescription says. You need to make these follow-up appointments for me. No, you can't take my PICC line out." I called the doctor and told him all of her concerns. He was so over it---"This woman is crazy. She has Munchausen Syndrome. She *needs* to be sick. She desperately needs psychiatric help. Anyhow, tell her that we did not adjust her Synthroid dose while she was here. Tell her she needs to follow up with all of those doctors listed. And her PICC line needs to come out before she leaves. Otherwise, she will use it for the wrong things and hurt herself."

Munchausen Syndrome. It rang a bell for me. It is a psychiatric problem. People create a bunch of signs and symptoms to appear ill. They like going to the doctor to get tests done. They usually know a good amount about medical conditions, terms, and treatments. They want to be sick even when tests show that there is nothing medically wrong. It's like they enjoy the attention of medical personnel. It made sense for this lady. She'd been to our hospital multiple times. She kept saying she had diarrhea when she didn't. She desperately wanted us to intervene when there was no need to. Very sad. She had a history of depression. Her affect was very flat and she seemed content to lie in bed all day and mope around. It was almost depressing to me. What really irked me and what always does about these kinds of patients is that they take time away from those who really are sick and need attention. Perhaps what was most peculiar about this woman's case was that she used to be a child psychologist. Even presently, she said that she volunteered as a victim counselor of some sort. Straaangge.

Anyhow, I finished gathering her discharge paperwork so that I could review it with her. I told the secretary as I headed toward the patient's room, "Alright, let me see if I can coax this lady out of here." Apparently the patient heard us at the desk. When I went into the room she said that she did not like us talking about her and ridiculing her. I felt a little bad honestly because I'm sure I had said some less-than-kind things about this lady (that she was off and had issues). I told her I was sorry. She didn't buy it but said, "This is a Christian hospital."

The woman did not want to leave us. She refused to have her PICC line removed and made a big deal about that. I had to get Pat involved. Eventually, I think she ended up going home with it. Anyhow, I made her paperwork look pretty, tied up loose ends on my part, and handed report off to the next nurse. Everyone wanted this lady to leave. She had no reason to be in the hospital any longer. I did my work and got her ready to go.

You'll find that psych patients are among the hardest to care for. And you'll see a lot of them, even if you don't work on a psych ward. Still, the general rules apply to them. Be kind, listen, etc. At the same time, be on your guard for manipulation, staff abuse, and patient self-harm. Do what you can to help them physically and in other realms. But these people really do need some focused psychiatric care and it's often hard for them to get it. Also, remember compassion. You don't know what this person has been through in her lifetime. Maybe she was a victim of sexual abuse or neglect. Maybe she had a difficult home situation. Sometimes you just don't know. Maybe some people are sort of jacked up by no fault of their own. *To a degree*, we are products of our environment.

Grossest Thing. People often ask me what's the most disgusting thing I've ever seen. To date, the answer is necrotizing fasciitis. Google that if you want to have nightmares. I took care of an older Caucasian female who was also very overweight. I can't remember her whole story but she'd had some sort of surgery for a wound she had developed. That wound had gotten infected and unfortunately, it was in her vagina and extended into her perineal area. It was a really unfortunate situation---she was on antibiotics and as a result, developed C-diff. As you can imagine, it was hard to keep that wound clean. I remember just thinking about how that wound was probably never going to heal. It didn't help that she was so large and could barely even move herself. Every time she defecated, her wound would get soiled. And it was a deep wound, one that could almost swallow your hand. Red and pink. Deep. Dirty. Smelled like poop.

I remember the day I had that patient. I also had three or four others and I remember all but one of mine were on isolation. I had to put a gown and gloves on before going in to almost every room. It's time consuming and really, it shouldn't have happened that one nurse would get so many isolation patients on her assignment. Especially on day shift. But I dealt with it. And fortunately, I had a great CNA helping me that day.

Most Rewarding Case. On the note of wound care, I think one of the most rewarding patients I cared for was a young guy. I believe he was late 20s, early 30s. He'd been out on St. Patrick's Day with friends and they decided it would be fun to light some things on fire. During their celebration, his arm caught on fire. He had some pretty bad burns, I'd say 2nd degree. He initially did go to the ER for treatment but then went back home. He came back and was admitted for IV antibiotics. I got to do his wound care. I gave him 0.5 mg Dilaudid beforehand. His fingers up to just above his elbow were burned. His outer layer of skin was gone. There was a yellow-tinged fluid where his skin had been.

The doctor was in the room when I removed the old dressing. I got to cleanse his arm with normal saline and clean off the old skin with gauze. Then I put some cream on it and covered the burns with Xeroform, I believe. Then we applied gauze and then wrapped it in Kerlix, a thin gauze that can be wrapped. It was a neat dressing change to do. This is the kind of work I think most people envision as "nursing."

I think the rewarding thing about helping that patient was that he was young. I am in no way an ageist. I really believe, however, that there is something awesome about helping young people. It's nice to know that the person still has a good 50 years or so to live. It's nice knowing that you're helping someone return to their job. This guy I think worked at the shipyard. He was also in school for engineering. It's so rewarding to help people get somewhere by restoring their health. That's why I chose nursing. You're extremely limited if you don't have health.

NG Tubes and Altered Mental Status. You'll quickly realize in your career how incredibly all-around draining/fatiguing/emotionally-stirring this job is. I cared for a patient who came in with chronic kidney failure. She was end-stage, in her 60s, and had come from a nursing home with altered mental status. I remember there were a bunch of wires hooked up to her head because neurology was monitoring her sleep waves and/or they were looking for seizure activity (I can't remember now). Anyhow, because she was confused and wasn't eating or drinking anything, the PA decided to order an NG tube---a tube that is inserted by nurses, through a nare and into the stomach. Placement is confirmed via x-ray.

The PA came in that day and put the order in for the NG tube near the end of the shift. I had to get this thing down, and it was the middle of my last med pass. It was very clear when I went into the room that the patient did not want this thing, as she shooed me away with her hands as I measured from her ear to her nose to her xyphoid process and explained to her what we were going to do. The aide was in the room with me as we went through this. Uhhh. The aide held the patient's hands down as I attempted to insert the tube. It was very clear that the patient did not want me to stick this tube up her nose. It was hard for the aide to hold her down. I didn't go too far. I explained to the aide that I was going to hold off and not force it. I told the doctor about this when he showed up; that the patient really didn't want this tube. He told me that it needed to be done.

The aide and I went back in the room for round two. She held the poor lady's arms down. I re-explained the procedure. Again, same situation as earlier. I proceeded to insert the NG tube up her nose. It always freaks me out when the tube hits resistance. I continued as the patient was herself resistant to this. Eventually, I got it to the back of the sinuses and down the throat. She started coughing and gagging. I told her to swallow, but she was neither cooperative nor coherent. She got teary-eyed and coughed profusely. The aide continued to hold her down. I remember my arms being up to try and tape down the tube once we got it in place. I felt the blood leave my hands and forearms. There was a very distinctive loud ringing in my ears. The room began to spin. I got lightheaded. I vaguely noticed the doctor come into the room (the one who's PA had ordered the NG tube). I simply said, "I need to sit down." I walked out of the room and into what seemed a different world. Fortunately, the nurses' station wasn't too far from the room I was in. I grabbed the closest chair, plopped down in it and kicked up my feet. "Whhheewww!", I said. A co-worker noticed me. I explained what happened. She jokingly asked if I was pregnant. The doctor came out shortly thereafter and asked if I was okay too. "I just needed to sit," I said.

Once I came back into reality and things got semi back to normal, I went back into the room. The patient had pulled out her NG tube. I know that if I had stayed in there much longer, I would have been on the floor. It was frustrating that after all that, she had pulled the tube out. So, I asked a co-worker if she'd help me. She did. I told her I'd pass some of her 5:00 meds if she'd do the NG tube for me. I sure as heck couldn't go through that again. She told me shortly thereafter that she'd gotten it down without much trouble. We ended up putting the patient in wrist restraints so she couldn't pull the tube out. The patient also had to go to dialysis. I ended up sending her to dialysis before the x-ray people could make it up to the floor to verify placement of the tube. Ooops. Not a huge deal, but my (more) experienced co-worker did inform me that I should have gotten the x-ray before sending the patient to dialysis. Oooopppps.

Later, in a non-related meeting with the interim-manager, I told her about what had happened. She said what I had experienced was indeed a near-fainting episode. Emotional stress is a cause of fainting. Yikes!

Dementia & Blood Draw. Another stressful experience I had occurred when I cared for an older lady with dementia. She was pretty out there. We had to move her close to the nurses station because she liked to climb out of bed and was a fall risk. Anyhow, it came time for the lab tech to draw her blood. She was having difficulty because of the patient's confusion. Both I and the clinical coordinator had to hold this poor little lady down so that her blood could be drawn. The patient's shrill scream pierced all of our ears. We had to close the door in her room so that she wouldn't disturb others. You'd think we were sawing the lady's arm off. We talked sweetly to her, though and tried to comfort her as she thrashed about and screamed while the small needle pricked her arm so that a blood sample could be drawn. Poor lady was crying. The lab tech was crying. It just took a minute or so but it was traumatic. Pat and I stayed for a minute afterward to comfort the poor lady.

Sudden Death. In this line of work, people die. That's just one more reason the profession is so stressful. Christmas day. I was sent to the ICU to help out. I was in the middle of bathing a patient when I got a phone call saying that my home floor got crazy busy so I had to go back there to help. Anyhow, in ICU, I worked with a very pleasant, thin, African American lady, who had COPD (Chronic Obstructive Pulmonary Disease). We got to talking a little bit and she was very nice. The following day, she was transferred to my floor because she was no longer considered so critical. That day, I helped her for a few hours. I had been in her room while rounding and saw that she was up in the bathroom. She had a steady gait and was fine to be up by herself. I went down the hall to do something in another patient's room. I heard Pat from around the corner (she has a voice that my ears seem to be drawn to; usually because what she says is so important). I heard her say loudly, "Somebody check on her! Somebody call a code!" I remember thinking Pat must have been in the tele room. She must have seen a slow heartbeat on the screen. I had a feeling it was my patient. That sudden strike of panic hit me in the heart and I was immediately aware of sympathetic nervous system. I ran out of the room I was in and into that little lady's room. There she was, lying lifeless on the bed, mouth open, eyes staring at the ceiling, when she had just walked to the bathroom minutes ago. It seemed unreal. How could she be dead? I was just talking to her!!

I heard the overhead system announce, "Code Blue, 3000 block." Everyone was rushing into the room—a few people had gotten there before me and had started chest compressions. In the mayhem, I remembered an important detail about this patient—she was a DNR (Do Not Resuscitate code status). "She's a DNR!" I almost shouted over the turmoil. "She's a DNR?" Yes! She's a DNR." I said it loudly several times. Even the hospitalist hadn't realized it. "Good job, Rebecca" he told me. (That made me feel really good because it came from one of my favorite doctors). We stopped our heroic efforts to try and restore the patient's heartbeat. "Cancel Code Blue, 3000 block" it said over the intercom. The crowd dissipated and I was left there, alone with my lifeless patient. I had later double checked the patient's chart to see again that DNR legal document with her signature at the bottom of it. In a strange way, it felt good to let someone go. To say it better, it was nice to know that we honored her wish. She was end-stage COPD and there wasn't much hope for her.

It really is bizarre, though, how fast some people go. Here one minute and gone the next. The spirit leaves but the body remains. It's strange. I almost couldn't believe she was dead. I remember touching her motionless body in search of a pulse. She *was* dead. No pulse. No respirations. No heartbeat. *Is she really dead?*, I thought to myself. Someone retrieved the post-mortem kit from the supply room. I and some other nurses and nurse aides worked together quietly and rolled the patient from side to side. We eventually got her body into the bag. We placed her patient ID sticker on the little cardboard-like nametag that came with the kit. The tag had a thin white string attached to it, which was tied around her cold big toe. Zip. A couple of us moved the now heavy bag onto a big cold gurney, which came from security on the first floor. We placed a sheet over her body. The scene was solemn. Quiet is suitable in these types of situations. It's respectful of the deceased. You'd hate to have an unexpected family member show up outside the room and hear a group of nursing staff chuckling and making jokes while working with your dead loved one.

    We wheeled the large gurney down the hall and into the private elevator. Down three stories. Again, down the long hallway, around some dark corners, through the automatic double doors. The security guard in his blue collared shirt met us just inside the double doors. He escorted us a little way. We stopped outside a heavy, locked door. The guard reached into his pocket and pulled out his keys, which were on a big ring. He told me to sign the book outside the door. Apparently, it was the book of death. I had to write the patient's name in it and then sign beside that my name with the date and time. I grabbed the pen with my right hand. The book was already open and when my eyes hit the page, I saw the long list of names written in different handwriting styles, which dated back a few months. The book was thick and full of names. It made me think about the book of Revelation in the Bible. I couldn't help but think about my name one day being in this book.

We proceeded to wheel the gurney into the now open heavy door. A dim light was on inside this small chamber, where there were several bunks to the left and the right. I looked and saw several other white body bags on some of the shelves. It was freezing inside. I tried not to breathe through my nose because I was afraid of the smell but nonetheless there was the scent of formaldehyde, which took me back to the cadaver lab in Dr. Stern's class. We were in fact in the morgue. And I'd been there before as a volunteer. I remember being shown see-through jars that had human embryos floating in them. Babies who never saw the light of day. There were several body bags in there back then too. I had been told it was people who were unidentified or unclaimed. They had no loved ones. The seemingly forgotten.

We lifted the stiff, lifeless body onto one of the bunks to rest alongside the others. *I hope someone keeps that heavy door open*, I thought to myself as we moved the body. We then stepped out of the crowded space. The light was turned off once we were out. I softly thanked the security guard for his time. The gurney was now empty and left in the guard's care. After all this I still wondered if the woman was truly dead. There was no pulse. My feet were aching and my body yearned to sit. My 13-hour day was finally over.

Similar story. On a normal day, I cared for a man who was in his 40s or 50s. Right off the bat, you could tell he was in bad shape because he was yellow. Jaundice. Not just in his eyes, but his skin all over was yellow. His liver was shot. A look into his history showed that he had abused alcohol. I took care of him on a Thursday. He was quiet. The day consisted of lying in a bed, breathing treatments every four hours, and morphine every few hours. I didn't work with him Friday because I was off. Saturday morning I noticed there were quite a few visitors in his room. He died a few hours later. He wasn't my patient that day, but I was asked by some co-workers to help bag his body. I removed the IV from his left arm that I had given Morphine through two days prior. I was cautious and wore gloves because I remembered that he had hep C. His body was still warm. His belly was distended. We rolled him back and forth respectively to get him into the bag. He was wheeled down to the morgue, the same place I'd taken the other lady a few months prior. In his room, we threw away some of the snacks that he'd eaten recently as well as some balloons and other personal belongings. It was sad. His room was cleaned and prepped for the next patient.

The longest code I've ever witnessed was in the ICU. We coded this one patient for I'd say over ½ an hour. I had floated to the ICU that day and heard "Code Blue 2700 block." It was the next unit over. I was so curious so I went down there. Apparently the staff had been expecting this guy to code. Codes in ICU are different than on the floor; they're less of a surprise there. I went into the room. I felt so helpless. One of the nurses asked me to hook up some suction equipment to the wall. The patient was a fairly large man. He was supine, his upper body exposed. The man had so many tubes going into and coming out of his body. The internist was already in the room; ICU has its own doctor most of the time. That day it was Dr. Raccoon, the pulmonary (lung) specialist. He was working on the patient like it was nothing. He seemed so comfortable. I just kind of watched. It was a neat experience. Sadly, the patient's loved ones were right outside the room. They got a glimpse of the resuscitation effort but the patient didn't make it. I inquired of one of the ICU nurses what the deal was with that patient, why he was so sick. Apparently he'd had some sort of bowel issue for which he'd had surgery. I believe he became septic and then spiraled downhill from there. I read his obituary a few days later. He was just in his 50s.

You'll see a lot of people die in your lifetime as a nurse, well, I guess mainly if you're on a medical floor in a hospital like I am. Hopefully that won't be the case if you're a pediatric nurse. Some deaths are expected and others are not. I've witnessed some unexpected ones and those are the toughest. I remember a lady in a nursing home I took care of. She wasn't even that old, 50s maybe. She ate her breakfast as usual that morning. A couple hours later she was pronounced dead. Being the young inquisitive person that I am, I asked the doctor later that day why the lady had died. The doctor said she didn't know but that the patient most likely had some sort of cardiomyopathy.

I remember another incident at the nursing home. I went in to check on a patient one night. I noticed she wasn't breathing (often times when I'm rounding I'll just swing by and stand at the doorway of a patient's room; if the patient is asleep, I'll just make sure I see a rise and fall of their chest. I know they're alive). Anyhow, this lady's chest did not rise and fall. I called her name. No response. I proceeded to tap her lightly, then more vigorously. I checked a pulse. Nothing. I left the room to notify the nurses. The patient was a DNR. They came in and we tried to check a blood pressure. No BP. The woman had passed---but peacefully. The doctor came by to officially say she was gone. We bathed her and cleaned her up, made her look presentable. The family was notified and a few people came to see her. Then eventually the funeral home people came to take her body away.

I've also watched patients die. That's a whole other realm. There's a very characteristic breathing pattern that they have when they're going. It's actually termed Cheyenne-Stokes. Often times you'll hear a deep breathing like the person is gasping for air. That'll be mixed with shallow breaths and a rattling sound. It's a weird phenomenon. Sometimes there will be pauses when the person doesn't breathe. To date, I'd say I've sat and watched maybe just two or three people die. One of these was a hospice patient that I went to visit at an assisted living facility when I was a hospice volunteer. The lady laid in the bed next to the windows that night. Every few minutes the nurse came in and dropped a few drops of morphine in her mouth to help ease any pain. I can't remember now what the lady had in terms of an illness. It was clear that she would die soon. I ended up leaving shortly before her death. A day or so later, I received a phone call from my supervisor. She told me that the medical/nursing staff at the facility thought highly of me. Word even got back to the patient's family that a volunteer had been there while their loved one was dying.

That's an experience that has always stood out to me. I think about when my grandfather was dying. He had an excellent nurse aide who was with him through his last days. I was fortunate to meet her. What a comfort it is and would be to know that your mother, father, grandfather, friend, or child didn't die alone. I think loneliness, especially in death, would be one of the worst things. But it touches my heart to hear about people who are surrounded by their loved ones when they die. The end of life is bitter. But, I encourage you to think about it, especially if you want to be a nurse because you will see it. And think about death for yourself. We're all going to meet it. What happens after we die? Is this all there is? If so, what a depressing existence. Believe me, I've thought about death a lot. And I'm convinced that there's more than this. It's ignorant to study the body—the chemistry, experiences, and elements that make us who we are and to say that in the end that's all there is. We as human beings are miracles. We are well-thought out, beautifully designed, and wonderfully created. If you just cracked open an anatomy book you'd understand that. There's no way we are a "mistake." I believe that this life is just the beginning. There's a hope worth living and dying for. There is a death in this life but I believe that there is also life or death on the other side. Through Jesus Christ, my soul will live on the other side. That life is available for all.

Whatever you believe, figure out why. Think about it. It will shape how you approach death. As a nurse, you'll see it and have to help others through it too. I truly pity those who believe this life is all there is.

Obituaries. On the note of death, one sad reality of nursing is that you will read about your patients in the newspaper. I've come across the obituaries of so many people I've cared for over the years, as both an aide and a nurse. It's disheartening. I've read about COPDers, really old patients, demented ones, and more. I think about their children that I've talked with. I think about the closeness I had to those patients—holding their hands, bathing them, feeding them, giving them medicine, and at times being the object of their rage during periods of extreme confusion. It can be depressing depending on how you look at it. I've been saddened when thinking about how hard I worked for nothing. The patient died in the end. My work was meaningless. Then you can think of it on a positive note. Maybe I helped make those last days comfortable for someone. Maybe I ministered to one of their kids or grandkids/other family member. Remember, your perspective matters. And in this life we may never figure out what kind of effect we've had on someone.

Blessing. I took care of a man who really ministered to me. He'd fought stage 4 colon cancer, was now being treated for cellulitis in a diabetic ulcer, had had skin cancer and some of his face taken off for it, had his back and knee messed up in a car accident, and now also had a pulled muscle in his abdomen. This man was smiling, laughing, and cracking jokes from the moment I met him.

I was amazed and slightly embarrassed looking back at myself, all the stupid stuff I complain about. Gee, it's hard waking up at 5:30 in the morning with my healthy body, driving my nice paid-for truck to work a job that I make good money in. All my prayers are answered. I'm healthy. I'm wealthy. I'm blessed. I lack nothing. I complain about silly silly silly things. And here's this man who has probably looked at death several times and yet he's rejoicing. Amazing. Your patients will minister to you. It's pretty cool.

Breast Cancer. Another patient who ministered to me: A 62-year-old lady. She had been to her primary care doctor to be seen for breast and arm swelling. She was given an antibiotic for a presumed infection. Over the following weeks, her symptoms got worse. She finally came to the emergency room after her husband told her to get checked out. The ER physician's note commented that he was concerned for malignant breast cancer. She was admitted to my floor. Blood tests for cancer markers were ordered, a breast biopsy was done at the bedside, and MRIs and ultrasounds were ordered to check for metastasis. They also put her on antibiotics in case there was any infection. I took over care for this patient shortly after she just found out about her most-likely unfortunate diagnosis. I spoke with the general surgeon who did the breast biopsy. She told me, "I'm 99% certain this is malignant breast cancer." When I looked at the woman's breast, it did have that classic textbook peau de' orange appearance seen with poor-outcome breast cancers.

I had entered her room just as the general surgeon was leaving. I introduced myself to her and asked her how she was. She said that her arm did hurt. I was able to get her some ice water and a Norco tab. I told her gently some of the side effects of narcotics since she'd never taken them before. I told her she could have Dilaudid if her arm still didn't feel better from the Norco. She and her husband both were so kind. He even smiled. She was sweet. My heart broke for them. I told them the plan from there forward without saying anything about a potential cancer diagnosis (I wasn't certain she had been told).

The quietness and kindness of this patient and her husband really marked me. I was overcome by compassion for them in their circumstance. I cannot imagine being in their shoes. I also couldn't help thinking about the woman's primary care physician who apparently overlooked this diagnosis. Her clinical presentation was very grim despite a normal mammogram the previous year. And her family history showed that both her mother and sister died of breast cancer. As I walked out of her room once, I placed my hands on her arm and said a quiet prayer that she would be healed. I really pray that this patient can be helped.

TLC Despite Rudeness. I mentioned maturity earlier, and here's a scenario that would have really bothered me a year ago but didn't this time around because I was able to view things from the patient's perspective. I cared for a 74-year-old man who had been treated for a non-STEMI. He had kidney problems too plus a history of BPH (Benign Prostatic Hyperplasia). Anyhow, from the moment I received report on him and all throughout the day that we interacted, all he seemed to do was complain. He talked to me for a while about how the hospitalist seeing him (i.e., one of my co-workers) was extremely incompetent. Later, that doctor and I spoke. I don't know what their conversation consisted of, but the doctor told me to give the patient some TLC (yes, Tender Loving Care). Good thing this is what we nurses are in the business of doing. The doctor wanted me to get this patient up and walking and check his oxygen sats. Physical therapy hadn't done it. I did it.

When I went in the room, the patient complained about the nursing assistant. It's sometimes hard to know what to do when patients complain to you about your fellow laborer. You don't want to throw your co-workers under the bus even if you think the patient is painting an accurate picture of your co-worker. Believe me, there's times where you will want to chime in and complain. But don't. I listened to my patient complain. There was even a time I went in while rounding and sat on the bedside commode (as a chair, not a toilet) that was next to his bed. I listened to him talk until the cardiologist came in. Some patients just want you to listen. When he complained about the hospitalist, I just told him, "Well, let's get you up and walking if you're in the mood. I'll make a note of it in the chart and the doctor will go from there." When he complained about the nursing assistant, I responded, "Well, we'll get it straight," referring to his O2 sats. This really was a patient who needed some TLC. We finally did get him up and moving. He did well walking and I told him that. I even complimented his beanie on his head. Later in the day, he told me, "You know, you're not as dumb as I thought." He even explained that he was trying to compliment me. He even said he didn't think nurses made enough money for their work. I'm so glad I was able to take a minute and just listen to this patient. I rounded on him. I sat with him. I encouraged him. Instead of trying to match his grumpiness on our first meeting, I tried to step back and see things from his point of view. He was sick. He was a DNR status. I'm so glad that I didn't snap back at him right away. God helped me to stay calm and not get frazzled. I'm so glad. I think it even helped my patient feel a little better.

The 14-Hour Day. I had just made it through a 14-hour day. I think it's actually the longest day I've ever had at my job. The previous one was back on that horrendous day I told you about earlier—not charting till 8:00 pm and going home and crying. Well, this particular day was very busy too, but I think I handled it better than I would have as a new nurse just off orientation. My day started with five patients, two of whom were on isolation and three who needed around-the-clock pain medicine. There was one other lady who needed pain meds too, but not as often. I had one patient on a heparin drip, two with cancer, one with a recent bowel obstruction, and the other with acute on chronic kidney failure. Luckily, I did have a CNA helping out and yes, four of the five were continent. Also, the group was together, not spread all over the unit. The IVCU nurses (they recover cardiac cat patients but help on the floor if work is slow for them) also helped me out some. Right out of the gate, after getting report from two nurses, I had four of the five patients asking me for pain medicine. Remember, the hard thing about pain meds is that you have to go back to the patient within an hour and reassess their pain. It's one of those things our hospital gets graded on, so to speak, for reimbursement. My morning med pass wasn't done until about 10:15.

I also had two patients with PICC lines, which meant I was responsible for drawing blood from them for lab. I did this three times throughout the day. I had a nephrologist ask to speak with me. A urine sample that he had ordered the day before on a patient had not yet been collected (I always try to please this doctor; urine specimen orders usually go overlooked and I know he gets frustrated with his orders not being seen, and also, he's a nice doctor). Granted, the patient was incontinent. I went into that patient's room to try and get the urine sample. PT was in there working with her, so I decided to try back. I did. I was able to help the lady, who was very weak, from her chair to the bedside commode. She started to urinate once on the commode. I let some trickle, asked her to open her legs, and then stuck the urine cup between her legs as she peed. Bingo. She'd also had a BM; I got a sample of that too, which had been also previously been ordered but not yet sent.

Anyhow, the day was busy mainly with meds and just trying to understand really what was going on with my patients. I didn't get a chance to read through charts like I wanted to. Reading patient charts is one of my favorite things about the job and it's great for learning purposes; it also helps you to better care for your patients if you actually know what's going on with them.

Five o'clock rolled around and I was in the middle of passing pain meds. My phone rang. "Rebecca, I'm going to give you an ER patient in Room 12," the charge nurse told me. "Is there any room closer that we can put the patient in?" "No, 17 is dirty"." "There's gotta be something closer, I'm all the way on the other end of the floor. How about 35?" "No, we don't get paid for putting patients in those rooms." "Well, okay, we'll aim for Room 17, but if the ER calls you have to tell them the room's not clean yet."

As I just barely came out of the room, someone at the desk told me that a patient's family member was on the phone and wanted to see how his mother was doing. Darn. This was the second time today he had called and I was tied up when he had called earlier in the day too. "Just tell him the patient's doing fine. I'm tied up right now."

Once I got out of that patient's room, I heard a call button and then "Are you going to help her?" asked a visitor/family member, referring to one of my patients in an isolation room that was trying to get to the bathroom. "Um, yes, I'm going to help her." I dropped whatever was on my mind and went in to help the patient get out of bed. She was a heavy lady who could walk with her walker. When she called to go to the bathroom, it meant she had to go right then. No waiting. She got to the toilet. "I feel nauseous." "Okay, I'll see if I can get you something for that." I told her I'd be back and to pull the cord for help when she was done. I bolted out of the room and all the way back to the main nurse's station to pull meds. As I was pulling meds, my phone rang, "Rebecca, ER is on the phone and wants to know if you've had a chance to look at the SBAR." "Ummm, I, I, I don't really have a choice. They're gonna bring the patient either way." "Tell them to bring the patient?? Okay." While I was talking on the phone, a fellow nurse tapped on the door of the med room. "Room 33," referring to the fact that the lady probably needed help getting out of the bathroom. I pulled meds on two patients but didn't even grab the nausea medicine for the lady in 33. I rushed back down to the other end of the unit where I had just been, dumped my pulled meds into a deep drawer at the nurses station (totally illegal), and then proceeded to go back into the isolation room and help this lady off the toilet. I wiped her bottom for her as she stood. She breathed heavily as we walked from the bathroom back to her bed. "I need...something...for...nausea." "Okay, I'll get you something here shortly." On the way out of the room, the aide told me that my patient in Room 36 needed pain medicine. Waaaahhhh!

This ER patient was on my mind. I knew I wouldn't lay eyes on her till almost shift change, as I had five patients to pass meds on at the other end of the unit. Dinner trays were also coming. Time for insulin too. My phone rang several times while passing meds, "Hey, the guy in 31 has a critical PTT value---180." "Oh, cool. We already D/Cd his drip." Ring ring. "Rebecca, your ER patient is here in 12." That call came around 5:30. I rushed around at the end of the floor I was on, finishing my med pass and trying to get everyone caught up on pain medicine. I made sure that my CNA had checked on the new patient in 12. Fortunately, she had.

I made my way to the nurses station in the middle of the floor (the main nurses station). The charge nurse said, "Oh, the patient in 12 is going to ICU." "What?!" "Yeah, she's obtunded, non-responsive. There's no bed yet in the ICU, though." I made my way toward Room 12 and finally got there by abut 6:35. I have to admit, I was actually relieved to see a quiet, sleeping patient with no one else in the room. I was afraid of the confrontation of a customer-service issue. I proceeded to assess the patient---

"Hello.??" There was no response. I rubbed her sternum, to which she barely opened her right eye. She had obvious left-sided facial drooping as well as some drool coming from her mouth. Someone had already put on her heart monitor, probably the awesome charge nurse. She had rhonchi in her lungs, a Foley draining clear/yellow urine, and 2+ edema on her feet. While in the room, I quickly pulled up her chart. A head CT had been done already before she came to the floor. It showed a "lacunar infarct," but it was unclear whether that was old or new. There was no sign of hemorrhage or lesions in the brain. I noticed that the doctor was still putting orders in for her.

The secretary came into the room and said, "Hey Rebecca, Dr. Aballah wants you to get a stat blood sugar on this lady." I did that next. It was 86. I reviewed some orders on this patient. A lot of her meds were due at 7 PM, which technically I was responsible for giving. The 2:30 dose of Levaquin was overdue from the ER. Had it been given? Did they get blood cultures on this lady? Urine? Where's she from? I searched through the chart to find some info on her, since I didn't receive a verbal/telephone report. Her history included lupus. My aide came in as I started to turn the patient. She helped me out. The patient had had a small BM. Her skin on her sacrum was intact. I wiped her bottom and put a Mepilex (a large band-aid like dressing that provides cushioning to bony prominences to help prevent pressure sores) on her sacrum. I left her positioned on her left side. I charted all this in a progress note. Seven o'clock rolled around. I saw that the assignment was still being created, so I decided I'd try to sort through some of the meds due in Room 12 and try to at least get them started for the next nurse coming on. I grabbed from the Pyxis: IV solumedrol, the overdue Levaquin, Zosyn, albuterol, IV protonix, and an aspirin suppository. When I got to the room, I realized I'd forgotten to grab the IV fluid. Back down the hall. Around this time, it was 7:15. I went ahead and gave report on one patient to a night-shift nurse. I headed back to Room 12 and bumped into the night shift nurse who was assigned to her. "Oh hey, Rebecca, can you do me a favor and call the nursing supervisor and see if they have a room for her yet? And if so, can you call report to the ICU nurse so we don't have to do report twice?" "Um, okay, I'll do that." I called the staffing office and got no response. I paged her and told the secretary.

I went back to Room 12. While sorting through her meds, I stumbled over her lab results drawn in the ER. Her potassium level was 6.3! Remember, the high end of normal is 5.5. A number this high could cause some serious arrhythmias. Well, I knew her heart monitor was on and I hadn't heard from the tele tech. I thought to check what her rhythm was, but didn't and decided to focus on trying to get some meds in her. "Albuterol. Why albuterol?," I thought to myself. "She's got no real respiratory distress." And then it hit me and I could clearly hear Dr. Winn's voice back from Critical Care days in school: "Kayexelate, certain breathing treatments, insulin…all of these can help treat hyperkalemia." Now it made sense. I checked back at the ER notes---the MD thought this patient also had pneumonia, which explained the Levaquin and Zosyn. Also, the ER nurse did make a note that Kayexelate had been given. While I proceeded to give meds, the night shift nurse I had just given report to came and stood in the doorway. "33's IV is infiltrated, so if you could look at that...Thanks." I had told him in report that her IV worked, her fluids were D/Cd, and she had been switched over to PO pain meds. I wasn't concerned about it and really wasn't going to do anything about it at that point. The look on my face must have made that clear, as the nurse didn't bring it up again even when I was handing over another patient to him shortly thereafter. I was able to get a few meds to the new ER patient in Room 12. Eventually the nursing supervisor called and said a bed was ready in the ICU.

    I scrambled and gave report to Gigi, the same night-shift veteran nurse who drilled me and made me burst out in tears when I had first come off orientation. I sat at the desk and gave her report on one of my patients from the day (we didn't do bedside report because she said she'd already been in and seen the patient. At this point, I wasn't concerned about doing things the right way with report, as it was going on 7:45 and I still had to hand off three other patients and transfer a patient to ICU. I gave her the scoop on the patient who had bladder cancer. I didn't know all the details of her history, but apparently Gigi expected me to know. She interrupts frequently in report too. "I sent her blood from the PICC line earlier this afternoon." Gigi said, "Pull up her labs." Her Hgb was 7.5. "Does the doctor know this?!" "I didn't tell her; this is the first time I've seen these results." "Well, are you gonna call him?" "No, Gigi, because it's almost 8:00!" She also asked me about the patient's JP drains, when I had last emptied them. "I haven't, but I will…" "I already did it." "Just make sure you flush her PICC line before you leave, okay?" I agreed in my head to do that.

    I know my loose ends were not all completely tied up before shift change, but on a day like this, I found it nearly impossible. My patients were all alive. They had all gotten their pain meds. The most important things of the day were done. Had I only had four patients all grouped together, yes, I would have tied up the loose ends. I did go back to that patient and say goodbye, flush her PICC line, and wish her a genuine "get-well."

    I went to the back nurse's station to call the ICU nurse to give report. I could almost tell by the tone of her voice that this wasn't going to go well. I gave her the best report that I could and told her I hadn't spoken to the ER nurse. She asked, "Has anyone charted an assessment on this patient?" "I did. It's in my Progress

Note." "No one's done the Admission Paperwork?" "No, she's not responsive, non-verbal, so I can't get anything out of her. She's from Coldman (a nearby nursing home), so I'm sure they have her information." Phone report was done.

After that, I sat at the desk and gave report to Eliza, a nice and new night-shifter. She could see my frustration and did not drill me during report. While we were in report, the phone rang. It was Gigi. Apparently she'd been talking to the ICU nurse I had just given report to and the ICU nurse had some questions. Eliza had answered the phone and was talking to Gigi who was talking to the ICU nurse. "Just tell her all that info is in my Progress Note (which is what I told her on the phone)." When we did go in the patient's room, the patient said she needed to be changed. I assured Eliza that my aide had cleaned her up right before shift change around 6:00. I had also hung a new bag of IV fluids to try to be courteous. Sometimes, you just have to point out the little things that you did do and try to focus on those. Eliza was so understanding and kindly told me to go home and get some rest. I was still a ways away from that.

After talking to Eliza, I gave report to yet another nurse on another one of my 6 patients. Yep, hand-off six patients to five different nurses. It doesn't get less efficient than that. That one went okay. Upon going into her room at shift change, that patient also asked for pain meds. I assured her she would get them soon from her oncoming nurse. I was trying to hurry through report because I wanted to get that one patient to the ICU and just simply go home. I'd had enough for the day.

Finally, back to Room 12. The charge nurse helped me wheel this patient down to ICU. I was so grateful. The night shift nurse on the floor who was supposed to get this patient also thanked me for transferring her. We wheeled into the ICU. I noticed the 2800 block, which has about seven or eight beds. There were no patients. The ICU nurse I'd spoken to on the phone got up from the desk and came to help us wheel the patient and move her onto the ICU bed. "What's her rhythm on the monitor?" "I don't even know," I said. "Her potassium's high. Did she get anything for that?" "I don't…" "They gave her Kayexelate in the ER," Jo, the charge nurse chimed in. She's good. As we got the patient on the ICU bed, the night shift nurse asked me in what I heard as "Half-ass, what are these fluids going at?," referring to the infusion rate of the IV fluids that were hanging. I stumbled over the answer as I pondered her spiteful address to me. *This is your ONE patient!!!*, I thought as I continued to assist with the patient. Of course, maybe she had TWO patients, but geesh. I had FIVE others upstairs plus this one critical one all the way on the other side of the floor, which is about five times the walking distance of the ICU. And this nurse was just coming on. The phone rang. The mean ICU nurse answered: "Oh, this patient's supposed to be in MRI? No, Rebecca's the day-shift nurse." It was the nursing supervisor. The patient had to go to MRI from there and had to be accompanied by a nurse. The ICU nurse looked at me. "I'm going home," I said sternly. It was 8:30 at this point. The ICU nurse said that she and the aide would take the patient to MRI. I did apologize for the messy situation. Jo and I left and went back upstairs.

In the elevator on the way up, Jo and I talked about staffing. We were both frustrated. Jo said that the ER has to whisk patients out of there quickly but that there's not enough nurses in the hospital to take these patients. This lady should have gone to MRI while in the ER, especially if there was concern of an acute stroke. Also, she should have never come to our floor in the first place, being so critical. There were no beds in ICU? The whole unit was empty? I suppose the hospital didn't want to open that whole unit just because of one patient. Remember, it's a money thing.

More Advice. Remember, on days like this, you just have to do the best you can. No, a tele nurse should not have six patients, especially when one is critical and she's on the complete other end of such a big floor from the other five patients. It is hard to know how much you need to do and at what point it's the next shift's job to do something. Believe me, I could have stayed there another 12 hours—perfecting my charting, trying to start an IV on the lady with the infiltrated one, passing pain meds in Room 32, providing incontinence care for the lady in Room 36, taking the ICU patient to MRI, and more, and there still would have been more work to do. And each of those nurse would have let me. I'm convinced that the ICU nurse would have let me do her job all night long.

Nursing is a 24-hour business. Do your best, but remember that there's always going to be more work to do. Short-staffing is a major problem in my workplace as I'm sure it is in the majority of places when it comes to nursing. I truly believe that nurses are underpaid and that poor staffing is a contributing factor to poor patient outcomes, poor patient satisfaction, higher hospital-acquired infection rates, and nurse burnout. Nurses cost money. Health care costs money.

Chapter 11: Dealing with Doctors

For all you new nurses, this is a good section for you. I've found in my first year of nursing that most of the doctors that I work with are pleasant and easy-going. Something that always bothered me in nursing school was hearing instructors verbally abuse physicians. I had one professor in general (whom I would deem a "lovey-dovey" liberal, feminist, typical college professor) who spent a lot of lecture time degrading doctors. She'd talk about, in a roundabout way, how many of them were incompetent and didn't like listening to women. Anyhow, to this day, it still really bothers me when I hear people talk about how rapacious doctors are---how they're out to get everyone, they're in it for the money, and they don't really care about people. My experiences with them have proven otherwise.

Because I'm on a med-surge floor, I've interacted with hospitalists, cardiologists, neurologists, vascular surgeons, nephrologists, infectious disease specialists, oncologists, and anesthesiologists. And yes, these names are intimidating and yes, doctors can make you feel stupid, but I've found that that's usually not intentional and more as a result of something I've done to myself. And I believe that doctors earn their money. They work long hours, sacrifice time with their families to help others, and spend a long time in school. They are trained. Keep in mind, however, that they are humans too. Yeah, they make mistakes. Society likes to put them on a pedestal, but at the end of the day, they are just like us. Here's some of my most memorable stories (both good and bad) involving doctors from my first year and a half of nursing.

I had a patient who'd had some sort of surgery that required her to get JP drains installed. I had emptied them throughout the shift. Again, you learn all those fancy words in school, like serous, sanguinous, serosanginous, etc. To this day, I still get them confused. The surgeon came into the room one day and interrupted what I was doing, just like most doctors do. He asked if I'd seen the drainage, how much of it, and what it looked like. I think I said it was a clear color. He responded, "So, it was serousssss drainage?" He seemed to emphasize the "s" sound. Now I'm not sure if that's how he talked or if he was trying to rub something in my face. I repeated back, "Serouss", with a little less emphasis on the s. This doctor reminded me of a lawyer or something. He carried himself like he was important. I told Richard the story that night when I got home. He thought it was hilarious. His response was that I should've asked the doctor, "Ssseriousssly? Serrroouusss drainage?" Hahaha! Again, have a solid support system. A sense of humor helps in this job too.

You'll have your share of snoody doctors in this line of work. It's unfortunate, but I guess in some way dealing with them makes you a better person. There's a number of ways to handle them. And also, you'll learn which docs are cool, which ones are patient, which ones are impatient, which ones prefer that you text-page them vs. which ones want you to call them, which ones you can actually understand and which ones are a little harder to understand because of their Japanese/Romanian/Indian/Spanish accents. Oh, it's a fun game.

There's one hospitalist that will hang up if you don't get to the desk within 20 seconds to speak to him on the phone. He's the same doctor who expects you to drop what you're doing and go with him into a patient's room or immediately stop what you're doing and right that second go walk the patient in the hallway and get their O2 sats, when it's really not that urgent and he could just write an order for it, which would allow the nurse to do it when it's most convenient for her.

And then you get doctors who don't want to put their own orders in. But then they'll get mad if you put their orders in for them because you've asked them three times to do it but they don't and then you end up putting it in wrong. We nurses have been told numerous times that we're not supposed to be putting orders in for the docs, unless it's some stat telephone or verbal order. It's quite irritating. You'll ask the doc for something, like IV Morphine, and he'll say, "Yeah, can you put that in?," even though he knows it's his job to do so and he's sitting right there at the desk. Or he'll tell you to put some order in and then by the time you get to it, the order set is different from the dose you're supposed to enter and you end up having to call the doc and wait for him to call you back so you can clarify the dose. But then if he's on hold for more than 20 seconds and you can't get back up to the desk in time because you're at the end of the hall in an isolation room cleaning up poop, the doc hangs up on you. Then the patient's all irritated because you still haven't delivered their pain med. Uuuuhhh, it's irritating.

You'll also run into some great doctors. Hang around them as much as you can. There's a cardiologist who comes to our floor who is awesome. He's of Greek descent but he's very easy to understand. He explains things very clearly and even puts orders in. He doesn't freak out when a patient is going downhill. He'll explain things to you. He even told me once, "If you have a question, just ask." One time I was really perplexed about the difference between Metoprolol (Toprolol) vs. Coreg for CHF. I ended up asking Tom, the cardiology PA. The first thing he said was, "That's a great question." He explained the difference to me very clearly—Toprolol is usually given if a patient has CHF and some sort of arrhythmia, like a-fib. Coreg is usually the number one choice for CHF without an arrhythmia because it improves the heart's ability to pump blood. It also has less effect on the heart rate. I had to jot down some notes on his comments. Another new nurse had the same question I had and I was able to share my findings with her.

Even if you're afraid to ask MDs questions, just subtly pay attention to when they prescribe things or do write orders. Always ask why when you're looking at meds. Look at trends in the patient's vital signs and read the doctor's notes. It'll explain some things to you. Most of the MDs I work with will list the patient's problems and then in the next column over, they'll list the treatment. For example:

Assessment/Problem (A/P):	Treatment
community-acquired pneumonia (CAP)	Levaquin q 24h, Solumedrol, breathing treatments PRN
Diarrhea	test stool for C-diff, dehydration
Dehydration	gentle IV fluids

Cough	Tussionex
a-fib, chronic	resume home meds-beta blocker, Cardizem

You can really learn a lot. Especially pay attention to the specialists' notes, like the nephrologists (kidney doctors), cardiologists, psychiatrists (on rare occasion), pulmonologists (lung specialists) and infectious disease docs. They know a ton and their notes reveal a lot. You'll get good at seeing patient problems via assessment and the chief complaint and being able to guess the subsequent tests, diagnoses, and treatment plans. It's really great training grounds if you want to go on to NP, PA, or MD yourself. Plus, it just makes you a better nurse because you can anticipate things.

I want to add something important on the topic of dealing with doctors. Never back down from them if you're doing something for a patient. Doctors all sound like they're in a huge rush because they probably are. But they'll speed through phone calls when you're trying to get an order for something. If you're on the phone with a doc and he's just given you an order for something and if you can't understand it because of his accent or a muffled line or whatever, politely let him know you're having difficulty understanding and request that he or she put the order in because you don't want to make a mistake. Let him know you're uncomfortable putting in an order that you are unsure of. This is one of the reasons we always do verbal readback. You say the patient's name (and should state their date of birth too) and read back the order that the doc gave you. State the drug, the dose, the route and the frequency of administration. Make sure that the two of you are on the same page. Don't let the doc slam the phone down without you verifying the order first. If he does, call him back. He'll probably yell at you but don't sweat it. Tell him you're following hospital policy and that you're ensuring patient safety, which really should be a top priority for every health care professional. He'll appreciate you reminding him of that. Patients have died because there's been confusion about orders. Always make sure that you and the doc are on the same page when he gives you a telephone and/or verbal order for something.

Oh, and procedures. I can't tell you the number of times I've heard patients say, "I didn't understand anything the doctor just told me." And this always seems to happen right after the doc has the left the room and the floor after attempting to explain an important procedure. Know that as an RN, it's not your responsibility to make sure the patient understands a cardiac cath or knee replacement or some other invasive procedure that a medical doctor is going to perform. It's the surgeon's job to do that. And this is why the docs should just take the informed consent paper into the room with them and get the patient to sign it right after they explain the procedure. It'd be nice if they actually informed the nurse that they were going to speak to the patient so that we could physically witness the doc speaking to the patient. But of course it never works this way in the real world. MDs tend to talk fast and then storm out of the room. A lot of times they will ask the patient if he or she has questions but I guess patients feel too overwhelmed or haven't had a chance to process the info in order to form questions. Patients usually think of questions that should be asked of the doctor once the doctor has left the floor. I think a better plan is that the patient get some reading/audiovisual educational material some length of time before the procedure and then the doc comes to explain it, and then the form is signed.

Nurses are not supposed to explain risks, complications, etc. of invasive procedures. Don't get caught up in this. If the patient is not prepared or has questions, let the MD know.

And when it comes to diagnoses/test results, etc., be careful. You can let patients know what they're H & H levels were for the morning and you can even read them the doc's notes. But, don't attempt to diagnose your patients. And be careful about disclosing certain results, like if a patient's recent labs indicate that he is hep C positive or that she does have HIV. That'll get you in a lot of trouble really fast. Some things are better said from the doctor's mouth. And sometimes as nurses we don't see the whole picture, so be cautious. Educate your patients as much as possible but let the doctor disclose big news, like cancer and such. Encourage patients to write their questions down and let them know that certain questions are for docs and not nurses to answer. Do explain medications and even wound care, etc. as much as you want. But don't diagnose, unless you've got the letters "NP" (Nurse Practitioner) behind your name.

One morning, I injured my elbow. It was a really cold morning. I was heading out the door a few minutes early to go heat my truck up before heading off to work (for a 12-hour shift, of course). I didn't realize that it had been so cold the night before. I ran out the door with my bags in hand. As soon as I stepped onto the porch, sllliiiipp. My feet went out from under me. I went up in the air and back down. All 125 pounds of me landed between a few chosen lumbar vertebrae against the sharp brick steps and my right elbow. I wish I'd had this accident on camera to look back on. I'm sure it looked like something out of a Looney Tunes episode. I was in shock by the fall and was well aware that it hurt, but I hopped right back up. I continued on to my truck. I went back upstairs and told Richard, "Be exxxxtreeeemelyyyy careful when you go down the stairs." We laughed about it later, but he felt bad that I'd gotten hurt. On the ride to work, I cried because my elbow was really hurting. I got concerned later in the morning when I noticed a tingly feeling in some of my fingers. It was also hard to move my elbow. I kept an ice pack on it as best I could. When the hospitalists rounded, I asked one of my favorite docs if she could look at it for me. I told her what happened and rolled up my sleeve. She assessed my elbow. She told me to take an ibuprofen and to ice it. She said if the swelling didn't go down that I should go get an x-ray. She said the swelling could be compressing a nerve, which could be causing the tingling sensation in my fingers. Fortunately, my elbow did get better. It meant a lot to me that Dr. Ray even took a moment to look at my elbow. She even asked a day or two later when she saw me how it was doing. Nice doctor. ☺

Another nice doctor story: In recently applying for nurse practitioner school, I needed to get some recommendation letters. I figured having one from a doctor would look really good. I typed up a recommendation letter for myself (yeah, I'd recommend me). I wrote it short and sweet---a summary of my work that Dr. MacGregor, one of the hospitalists I worked with could attest to. I handed it to him one day when he was at the computer and told him what I was going for. "I've already written this recommendation letter for you. Do you mind signing it for me?" He could see that I'd even typed his name at the bottom of the letter. "You're smart," he smirked. "I think you do a great job here with our patients."He skimmed the letter over and with a few squiggles, signed his name. "Good luck," he said. I thanked him and then came back to him a few minutes later with a bag of mixed chocolate truffles. I had heard a fellow nurse say that he liked chocolate.

Now, I have to say that I do feel quite privileged to be able to work with doctors. Who else gets to work so closely with such knowledgeable people? And they have practical knowledge. Useful knowledge. I love learning from them. They are great resources.

I always like to pick the brains of doctors. One day I spotted Dr. A at the back nurses station on the unit. He was charting. I started up a conversation with him. (Mind you, this is the same doctor of the "serrrouussss" story I shared earlier). I asked Dr. A a question: "Do you ever regret that you chose medicine?" He told me simply, "No, I don't. I love what I do." He elaborated. "I have two sons, though, and I discourage them from going into medicine." He told me that medicine has changed a lot from when he first started out. He said he spends a lot of time on paperwork, nearly as much as he spends with patients. He said he works long days. He did, however, say that the outlook for nurse practitioners is pretty good. He encouraged me to get some ICU experience and even told me to feel free to call his office in order to speak with their nurse practitioner. I told him that I had thought about medical school at one point in time. He sighed when we brought up the cost of med school, again, another reason he discouraged his young sons from becoming doctors. It's always neat to get a doctor's perspective. I also appreciated his advice.

On a Sunday morning, I was half asleep. It was day 3 in a row for me. I was exhausted. A physician had come to the floor and was cursing and ranting and raving about how pathetic ICU nurses were. His patient who had had some vascular bypass surgery done was now on my floor. He was upset because her surgical dressings had not been changed. When I had received report on the patient the day before, there had been no mention of dressing changes. And I've always been told that nurses should never touch surgical dressings—the surgeon always does the first dressing change after surgery. They're very intense about that kind of stuff. Don't touch a surgeon's stuff. This woman's chart revealed no orders for dressing changes. The surgeon was very upset that his patient's dressings had not been changed. *If you want something to be done, doc, you gotta put the orders in,* I thought to myself as I heard him nearly screaming obscenities. I don't do things without an order from the doctor, especially surgical dressing changes.

This patient also had some issues with urinary retention. He wanted me to bladder scan and insert a Foley if necessary. He gave some verbal orders for dressing changes. I went downstairs to get the bladder scanner and then came back up. I repeated to him what he had told me to do for the patient's dressing change. "No, it's..." I repeated that and he was satisfied. It was a simple task. I wanted to make sure I fully understood. "I'll go ahead and do the dressings now," I told him. I gathered supplies while he sat at the desk. I spent a long time in the patient's room, doing her dressing changes and a bladder scan. Turns out she did need a Foley, so I put one in. I changed her dressings just as Dr. South had asked me to. He was happy at the end of all of it. I was happy he finally put written orders into the computer. It was almost humorous to me that he got so upset. *Dude, just put the orders in if you want it to get done*, was all I could think. It seemed to me that he had some deep-seated problems with ICU nurses. He seemed to think they didn't do anything. I actually do like this surgeon, despite his little tirade.

I told Richard this story when I got home that night. He got upset thinking about a doctor cursing at me. I told him, though, that I think the doctor was more cursing *to* me about other nurses, rather than *at* me. Richard gave me some tips on how to handle that---"Doctor, you're not gonna get anything out of me by talking to me like that. You're being unprofessional and you need to calm down. I'm going to call Human Resources and report your behavior. I'm here to listen when you're able to talk to me with some respect." Easier said than done. Richard has much more of a backbone than I do, but I'm learning. Fortunately, the situation wasn't too bad, but it was just a little bit uncomfortable. Perhaps I can use Richard's advice the next time something similar happens.

Another doctor I work with frequently is an interesting guy. He's nice. It's funny to me, though, some of the stuff he does. It frustrates me, the way he acts toward nurses at times. He acts like he's in a hurry and really busy but disregards the fact that nurses are just as busy. He often comes to the front desk. He'll pull up a patient's chart in the computer, swivel around in his chair, and loudly say, "Who's the nurse for Ms. Jones in Room 3018?" He expects everyone at the desk to stop what they're doing and exhaust all means to get that nurse up to the front desk as soon as possible. It's funny to me that the secretary will call the nurse as will a few other nurses. Some people even go on foot to look for the nurse that the doctor needs. I know I've done it. I know I've been tied up with something intense like wound care or I've been in the middle of inserting a catheter in an isolation room and I've had to leave, run all the way to the front and walk with this doctor to another patient's room, take a bunch of verbal orders, and be expected to do them immediately.

 I have, however, learned another trick from Richard in dealing with this doctor (and just all people in general). I was amazed at how well it worked when I applied this technique. This doctor caught me in the hallway when I was walking back and forth from a patient's room. I was in the middle of something and really trying hard to get it done for the patient. On my floor, it's very difficult to do anything that takes 10 solid, uninterrupted minutes in one shot. There's just a lot of interruptions. Anyhow, I was really focused this time around. This doctor asked me, "Oh hey, I need you to walk this patient in the hallway for five minutes and record their O2 sats and heart rate for me." "Oh, okay, walk and record O2 sats and heart rate. You know, give me about 10 minutes; I'm in the middle of working with this other patient but I will get on that as soon as I'm done over here." When I was finished with my task, I went to go do that thing for the doctor. He had already done it himself because he didn't want to wait five minutes. I was so amazed!

The trick here is to show other people that you are legitimately busy (it bothers me when people don't realize how busy nurses are). If you tell the person asking you for help that you will be with them shortly (5-10 minutes, or even longer---give them a time frame), a lot of times, they will end up doing it themselves or asking someone else for help because that route is quicker. It's awesome. Again, this is not a way to avoid helping people. But it is a great tool to use if you feel that people don't appreciate the value of your time.

I also felt slightly thrown under the bus by this doctor. I had called him asking for pain medicine for a patient. I paged him several times but did not ever receive an order for pain medicine. I can't remember the whole story here; I think it was just that my page wasn't returned. Anyhow, I had been pestering him for some time about getting this patient some pain medicine. When he finally showed up on the floor to round, he called me to walk into the patient's room with him. "Oh, so you've been having some pain, huh?" Patient: "Yeah, I've actually been in a lot of pain and I just wish we could do something about it." Doctor, turning to me, still standing in front of the patient: "Hey, I definitely want to know when my patients are in pain." Whhhaaaattt???!!! The way the doc said this to me right in front of the patient really made me angry. I had been nagging him for a while trying to get pain medicine for the poor guy and then he made it look like I hadn't done anything and that he was completely unaware of the patient's condition. Uuurrrr. Remember what I talked about earlier---let your patients know when you call the doctor to try to get pain medicine. At least it shows them that you're advocating for them, even if the doctor doesn't think so.

Another doctor I work with, I'll call her Dr. D, is an interesting lady. She is very fashionable and speaks fluent Spanish. She's a native of the Dominican Republic. Her English is slurred, which makes her difficult to understand. Anyhow, I took care of one of her patients who had some psychiatric issues. This patient was being discharged from our hospital and was being sent to a psych center. Any time a patient is discharged from our hospital to another facility for treatment, for whatever reason, we have to fill out a form called "EMTALA---Emergency Medical Treatment and Labor Act" (see www.acep.org). It's a nightmare to do the paperwork for this thing. It is time-consuming. Thank you, federal government. A lot of people, including the patient's primary nurse, the physician, and the nursing supervisor have to fill out a section of the form. Fortunately, we don't have to do it very often. Anyhow, I had Pat help me fill out my section of the form so that it would be done by the time Dr. D came to the floor. Pat, the one person who does know how to handle EMTALA, assured me that my part was complete up to the point that I could fill it out (I still did not yet have the name of the nurse who would be receiving the patient).

When Dr. D came to the floor, she had expected that I would have completed her section of EMTALA as well as my section. "Why is your part not done?! I cannot see it on my computer." I assured her that I had filled out my section. "This is supposed to be done! Do it (insert Hispanic twang)!" I tried to call Pat so she could come explain to Dr. D how to do her portion. As I was at the desk doing other paperwork and trying to hunt down Pat to help Dr. D, Dr. D snoodily looked at me and said, "Were you waiting until I got home to call me and tell me to come back and fill this out?!" Man, I wanted to give her a piece of my mind— *Woman, you make X amount of money and you don't know how to fill out your portion of this form.* It's not my job to fill this out for you!!!" Urrr, she made me angry. I think I was just really frustrated again, at the government's involvement in health care and the fact that I was trying to deal with this five minutes before my shift was to end. Pat finally showed up and basically filled out Dr. D's portion for her. She's so good at handling situations like that. Another very nice hospitalist I've worked with knows how to fill out his portion and it is a smoother process.

Another rude doctor I dealt with was Dr. G. He rarely comes to our floor, but had come up one day to do a small procedure at the bedside. Dr. G is a podiatry surgeon---he focuses on foot problems. I recognized him because of when I had volunteered in the same hospital several years prior; I spent one day shadowing in his office. My interaction with him was frustrating this time around. I had just left a code and was heading into the medication room to pull dextrose, insulin, and Kayexleate for a patient of mine (the same guy from one of the PainFULL patient stories) who had a high potassium level. He was end-stage renal. I had been interrupted by the code the first time around when I tried to deal with his hyperkalemia. The hospitalist had even explained his written orders for me to make sure I dealt with this properly. The same hospitalist was in the code where I had been and told me, "We need to get that other patient's potassium down so we don't have another code." As I entered the medication room to pull the meds for this patient, I noticed that the door didn't shut behind me. It was a man in a sweater and khakis. No ID was visible. "Can you get me some lidocaine, gauze, such and such needles, and etc.?" I stopped what I was about to do and searched for his supplies. I tried to direct him to the secretary for help but instead ended up walking him to the PAR room where we keep supplies. Apparently our floor didn't have everything he needed. "Whenever I come to this floor, y'all never have what I need, so why do we do this procedure at the bedside?" I was totally uninterested in what he was saying because all I could think about was my patient with the high potassium level. I can't remember what happened; I think eventually I hooked him up with the nurse who had his patient.

Later, I was at the desk still charting things related to the hyperkalemia patient when Dr. G asked me how to put orders in for a type of test he needed done. Urrr, another doctor who didn't know how to put orders in. I was patient with him and helped him. I even called the lab for him to find out exactly how to place the order. I did all of the things he should have done for himself. Just to vex him a little (bad, I know), when I placed the order in the computer I said, "You're Dr. Graham, right?" "No! G," he stated back to me. "Okay, it's done." "Thanks."

Looking back, and after telling this story to Richard, I learned how I should have handled this situation. I should have asked to see his ID, since he really could have been anyone. Besides, hospital staff are supposed to wear their badges above the waist, where they are easily visible. Since I was really in the middle of something very important---treating hyperkalemia, with verbal and written orders from a doctor when I was interrupted by this doctor who was not seeing one of my patients, I really should have told him, "Um, sir, hospital policy is that you are not supposed to interrupt nurses while they're pulling meds---it can cause fatal errors. Let me finish here and I'll be right with you." Just with that, I should have shut the door. He likely would have found some other poor nurse to pester instead of waiting for me. (Remember, if you tell people to wait 5 or 10 minutes, they usually find another way to get things done). If he waited, I should have directed him to the secretary to have her call the patient's nurse so that she could have dealt with the issue. I could have told him right off the bat, "I'm in the middle of something very important; this patient could die if I don't take care of this right now. I'll be with you in about 20 minutes, once I'm done resolving this issue." Again, he would have found some other way to solve his problem. Also, I could have just told him to call the lab by giving him the number and letting him ask how to put his orders in. Then he'd know for next time.

Always be learning. Take awkward doctor interactions and learn from them for next time. Believe me, you'll have plenty of them.

Chapter 12: Charge Nurse

At this point in writing, I've been at my job nearly two years. I can say that I have had some charge nurse experience (maybe only about seven or eight days-worth). Charge nurse experience is a great thing to get under your belt. The charge nurse is responsible for a lot of things---you check the code carts to make sure they're working, you check the medication refrigerators and food fridges and freezers to make sure they're operating right, you assign patients to nurses as transfers and admissions and discharges come and go. You make sure the floor nurses on your unit have the supplies they need; if not you call the nursing supervisor to get it, you make the assignment for the next shift, you help with any issues that arise, you help your floor nurses with anything they need, sub-in for the tele tech when she goes to lunch, answer phones and call buttons, make sure people are following up on Quality-Control charting, etcetera. It's a lot of responsibility for only an extra dollar an hour. And you're either free charge or Resource. Resource means you are the charge nurse but that you also have a patient load yourself. This is very difficult, as you can imagine because it's hard to know what's going on with other patients when you have your own to look after. Free Charge is awesome on the other hand, at least in my opinion. Free Charge means you don't have patients. I got to do this for the first time on a Sunday and it was great. I went around helping with vital signs and anything else that people needed. As you can imagine, I still stayed busy, though.

The most important thing as charge nurse is to try to know how your teammates are doing. Since you make the assignment for the next shift and since you assign patients to nurses, you don't want to overload a nurse who is already drowning by giving her another heavy patient. Look out for you co-workers. See if they need help passing meds or calling a doctor or starting IVs. Make yourself available. Be cautious in this too, though, because you can still become overwhelmed yourself.

Charge nurse, at least on the weekends, is like being the clinical coordinator. You are essentially, in charge. If someone gets angry and wants to "talk to wherever's in charge," it's you. You'll also work with the staffing office and maybe even administrators. So be alert. Be on your toes. You'll quickly learn that holding this role or title means serving. I've really learned this from my clinical coordinator and some managers. The higher up you get, the more of a servant you are. It's a lot of responsibility.

Chapter 13: Final Closing

Why Nursing is Great. It may seem like I've spent a lot of this book complaining. I am trying to be realistic, not necessarily discourage you from going in to this line of work. I do want to make it clear, though, that nursing is *not* for everyone. There are excellent doctors who would make horrible nurses. There are pharmacists that shouldn't be nurses. But nursing is, for a number of reasons, a good field to work in. It *is* for some people. Occasionally you'll run into a nurse who seems to have been made for nursing. I recently came across a coffee mug online that said, "I'm a nurse, what's your superpower?" It made me laugh. Nursing is not for the weak. It will try you. It will demand your brain, your thoughts and intellect, your emotions, your heart, your soul, your compassion, your empathy, your love. It requires a lot, yet it also offers so much in return.

Perhaps the greatest thing about nursing is the human interaction. In what other job do you get to be so close to another person? You, whether you want to or not, learn about another human being's socioeconomic situation, his home life, his past, his job, his education. You learn about his family, his heartbreaks, his toughest trials and greatest triumphs. You hear each person's story. And as a nurse, you become a part of it. You have a part in the healing process. You play a role in giving people their lives back. You get to make people comfortable on the worst day of their lives. You get to put a hand on their shoulder, give a hug, hand a tissue, offer a hot cup of coffee, cover someone with a warm blanket. You get to administer life-saving medicine. You get to watch over them, like an angel would. You protect them from the overworked, rushed, stressed out doctor or pharmacist by acting as that last checkpoint in the treatment process. You make sure the patient is safe, even if no one else does. You are that person who steps aside, who goes under, who does what needs to be done to help the patient in the worst of scenarios. You get to smile and laugh and share good news. You get to see the good that comes from a cardiac cath when a blood vessel is reperfused, a baby is born, a heartbeat is revived after CPR, a stroke patient walks again, a patient breathes better after bronchodilating drugs are given. You relieve pain. You help bring life. You help restore life. You offer people a second chance. You become a friend to the friendless; some days you'll be the only one to enter a patient's room (other than a 30 second visit from the doc). You'll be there, when no one else is. You *SHOW* love and compassion. You *show* people that they are not alone. You show them that they are valuable.

In nursing, you get to learn about so many things in the human body. You learn the basics of anatomy and how each human body is built quite similarly, but yet you also quickly learn that not every body is exactly the same. You also get to learn about how we're all genetically different. You learn about disease processes—how they start and take over. Then you get to learn about a myriad of fascinating medications, their make-up, and how they interact in the body to heal people. It's amazing. You'll be in awe when you think about the people who make drugs. They're brilliant. As a nurse, you get to be in the middle of a lot of great professions, so you sort of luck out all around. You get to bounce ideas and questions off of doctors, hear why pharmacists recommend a PO (oral) form of a drug over the IV (intravenous) form, and how psychiatrists conclude whether someone is mentally ill or not. It's so fascinating.

In the world of nursing, the ceiling is tall. You can always learn more. And that means formal education as well as non-formal. Even just with an associate's degree, you can do a lot. With a bachelor's you can do a little more. You can be a manager if you want. That bachelor's degree sets you up to get a master's degree—as a family nurse practitioner, a nurse anesthetist, a nurse midwife, a geriatric nurse practitioner, a nurse educator, and a host of other things. Even with the smallest nursing degree, you can work in so many different areas. There's orthopedics, oncology, cardiology, neurovascular, operating room/surgical nursing, emergency/critical care nursing, rehabilitation, labor & delivery, mother/baby, pediatrics, school nursing, occupational health nursing, and on and on. You can work in a hospital, a nursing home, a rehab center, another person's house, a school, on a boat, or in a doctor's office. There is so much to choose from. Typically, if you don't like one area, try out another. Few nurses stay in one area throughout their entire career.

One last thing on why nursing is great: It makes *you* a better person. Despite the fact that we are all disgusting, sinful, evil creatures, I believe that all human beings are capable of good. Nursing is a world of good. On days I work, I very rarely think about myself. In the midst of running around helping patients go to the bathroom, doing dressing changes, reading charts, starting IVs, hanging antibiotics, organizing my day, and performing one of the other many tasks asked of me, I somehow forget about why this month's water bill is $300 or how long Richard and I will have to share one vehicle because his is in the shop (first world problems, I know). I don't have time to dwell on some embarrassing thing I said or did the day before. I forget about my Facebook status, my weekend plans, and what I'm going to eat for dinner. My attention is fully on the needs of other people. Also, being a nurse makes you very happy that you're not a patient. You realize that in the grand scheme of things, you're not the one lying in a bed, in pain, unable to move or speak or control anything around you. You suddenly realize that you don't have any problems or reasons to complain.

Another reason nursing is great is that you can really make a difference. If you think something needs to be changed, if something can be better or more efficient, or if you feel like a new system is needed, do something about it. It's so funny; one night I came home really frustrated and I told Richard about it. He asked me so nonchalantly, "Well, why don't you guys just have something that…?" I'm leaving it blank because I don't want to give away an idea. Anyhow, his simple question to me has led us to pursue a U.S. Patent for an idea that would greatly improve nursing workflow and patient/family satisfaction. I never thought we'd be on this track.

Think about specialty beds, chest tubes, bedpans, urinals, and all the other cool gadgets in this field. Somebody wanted to solve a problem or make things a little bit easier or better for themselves and others. As a nurse, you are at the forefront of patient care. You know what patients need. You know what they want. You know what you and your co-workers and bosses want. You often know what works and doesn't work. I encourage you to think about or take note of all the things that bug you about your job. Think of all the little things that aggravate you because they're so complex. Is there a way to simplify? Is there a way to improve workflow and make things quicker, safer, or more enjoyable? If you think so, do something about it. That's why I'm writing this book—I wanted to help prospective nurses, nursing students, and new nurses. I want to share my experience.

Read. As a new nurse and just a nurse in general, I encourage you to read. Read the stories of sick people. One of the most touching books I've ever read was shortly after I started working—Christopher Reeves' book titled *Still Me*. He talks about the nurses who made a difference for him. Imagine taking care of Superman. His story is tragic, the accident that is. But it is also inspiring and motivating. He did not curse himself and give up such a hard fight. He fought and still accomplished so much good although he was confined to a wheelchair. He raised awareness about spinal cord injury. He shared his story. He didn't let a tragic accident and wheelchair confinement stop him. He was still Superman, just in a different way.

Another good read is *The Diving Bell and the Butterfly* by Jean-Dominique Bauby. It's the story of a newspaper editor who suffered a massive stroke at the brainstem. He developed a way of communicating with his nurse so that he could share his story although he could not speak or express emotion other than with the blink of one eye. Remarkable.

Read to try to understand others' stories. Imagine if you were a prisoner in your own body. Imagine being paralyzed. Imagine a tube in your throat, being on a ventilator, being in chronic or severe pain, being unable to communicate. Try as much as you can to understand other people's points of view. It'll make you a better nurse. I realized while reading Christopher Reeves' story and the other patient's story that my life really isn't that hard. I'd pick my job and my life and the "difficulties" of my job any day over being a patient. I often tell people, "The more I'm a nurse, the less I ever want to be a patient." Being sick is no joke. It takes your life from you.

And again, that's why I'm a nurse. To prevent illness, to bring hope and healing, to give people their lives back. I encourage you to take what's been presented here, my experiences and my story and thoughts, and ask yourself what you want to do. Now that you know what nursing is *really* like, is it for you?

At the time I started writing this book, I thought it would simply be a collection of stories from nursing school and my subsequent first year in the real world. However, it is hard to limit my collection of stories to just the first year. Right now, I am at nearly the two year mark at the same job I started in. So much has happened and I have grown tremendously as a person and as a nurse, so I have to include stories up to this point. It's interesting to look back and say, "Oh wow, remember this time a year ago when I was in this situation. I wouldn't have known what to do; I would have been so overwhelmed." Or "This time last year, I didn't have this certification" or "I didn't know that last year." Nursing has taught me so much. I've certainly matured as a person too. I know I'm maturing when I've ceased to be so easily offended and I can first think of other people, not myself.

Next month will mark two years I've been an RN on a tele floor. I learned last week that I've been admitted to a family nurse practitioner (Master of Science in Nursing) program. I'll start in the fall and be full-time. I plan to still keep a foot in the door and stay PRN where I'm at now. I've tried jumping ship; last year when work really started to put me down, I put in about 25 job applications elsewhere. I had three interviews but no offers. I really think God's kept me where I'm at for a reason. And believe me, I've seen a lot of nurses come and go. Turnover is very high where I'm at. But I do believe that there are benefits of putting roots down. My employer has been good to me---I've learned so much, gotten a great start in nursing, gotten paid time off, been able to make a living while out of my parents' nest. And through writing this book, I'm able to share my experiences with other potential nurses.

Nurses are vital to the health care community. They are the ultimate patient advocates. They are the laborers, the human face and human touch in a scary place. And while nursing is not as glamorous as it may seem—with bedpan duty, feeding patients, and even changing linen, it is also practical—elevating the head of a bed for a patient in respiratory distress, knowing that a patient is about to tank based off of early warning signs, intervening early through assessment and medication administration. It is providing life-saving medical care. It is helping patients take the next step. It is connecting them to resources.

The world needs good, competent, caring nurses. It also needs nurses that are not overworked—verbally and physically abused, underpaid, and stretched thin. Administrators, managers, and even government officials need to look at nurse burnout. It's not good for anyone.

Nursing as a career, as challenging as it can be, is worth it. Remember, though, it is not for everyone. It will demand a lot of you, more than you have to give. If you choose to take this path, do it for the right reasons. Know that it's not about you. Do it to help others and to make their lives better. If you push through the awkward encounters, the trying days, and all else, I'm sure you'll come out a better person as well. I hope you have found this book helpful.

Your Invitation. To answer the question of how we fix the problem of humanity, there is one answer. Jesus. As a nurse who is a follower of Jesus Christ, I am mindful that I am His hands and feet everyday that I walk into my workplace. If you read the

Gospels, Jesus was drawn to the types of people in need of nursing services—the sick, the lame, the poor, the sinners. He despised arrogance. We're all called to follow Him. We were made for His good pleasure. I am supposed to minister to these people I encounter. Perhaps by living my life and by practicing what I believe…loving God, pursuing Him, being in fellowship with Him, knowing His Word, speaking life, loving people, giving medicine, cleaning up excrement, feeding a patient, loving my husband, etc., I can encourage someone else. Nursing is a wonderful platform for that. It's ground zero for making the world a better place.

I believe in the power of Jesus Christ to save people from themselves and from hell. The Bible, God's Word, provides instruction on everything we need to know to live this life effectively in order to please God, for whom we were made. Without Jesus, there is no compassion. Without Him, there is no salvation, freedom, morality, redemption, justice, patience, love, humility, joy, goodness, or faith. The world needs Him. It needs to see His love. Relationship with Him is the answer. Everything flows from that.

The salvation He offers is for ALL people. It doesn't matter what you've done. It doesn't matter what you haven't done. Turn away from yourself and to Him. Without His help, it's hard to be a good nurse, and not to mention, impossible to get into heaven. If Christ is not living in you, I encourage you to welcome Him. His arms are open wide and His heart is full of love and mercy for you. If you're skeptical, check out some Apologetics books – *The New Evidence That Demands a Verdict* by Josh McDowell and *Jesus on Trial* by David Limbaugh. What do you have to lose—eternal life?

Romans 10: 8b-13 (Holman Christian Standard Bible): "This is the message of faith that we proclaim: [9] If you confess with your mouth, "Jesus is Lord," and believe in your heart that God raised Him from the dead, you will be saved. [10] One believes with the heart, resulting in righteousness, and one confesses with the mouth, resulting in salvation. [11] Now the Scripture says, Everyone who believes on Him will not be put to shame, [12] for there is no distinction between Jew and Greek, since the same Lord of all is rich to all who call on Him. [13] For everyone who calls on the name of the Lord will be saved." Call on Him today.

APPENDIX

Here you'll find a collection of my work—papers and pre-clinical paperwork from nursing school. I have included grading rubrics/evaluation forms at the end of them so you can get an idea of what the instructors use when grading you. A word to the wise when it comes to writing papers for nursing school: Follow the grading rubric. The closer you to stick to it and give the instructor what she wants, the better your grade will be.

Please also note that some of the formatting of these papers has been changed from their original formats. Be sure that you learn APA (American Psychological Association) format or whatever format it is that your school uses for papers. Follow the rules for spacing, content, formatting, and everything else.

Rebecca Parker

Personal Philosophy of Nursing

Fall 2010

My least favorite part of nursing school thus far is spending 3 hours of my Friday afternoons sitting in a class on nursing "theory." If someone else's beliefs or theories have not been proven to provide some distinct advantage in the real-world, why is there a need to learn about it, not to mention, implement it in my practice? Each person has his or her own theory for everything under the sun, so I will attempt to articulate my own personal philosophy of nursing; that is, my own set of beliefs and opinions that shape my thought process, which later guides my actions (Johnson & Webber, 2010). Perhaps in the process of exploring my own beliefs about this profession, I will be better able to serve as a registered nurse.

Personal Philosophy of Nursing

I remember as a 9-year-old girl reading a book about Clara Barton, founder of the American Red Cross. She served during the Civil War as a nurse on the front lines aiding soldiers who had been injured (American Red Cross, 2010). The black-and-white sketches in the book and the author's descriptive words created in my mind the image of a real nurse—compassionate, kind, and competent; someone in the middle of the action, the one keeping things going by saving lives, healing wounds, and meeting a host of other needs for those in her care.

Although it may sound cliché, I believe that nursing is a way of life. Nurses actively pursue knowledge. They define empathy and compassion. They treat their patients how they would wish to be treated if the tables were turned. Nurses act with integrity, causing no harm to those entrusted to their care. They serve hospitably and responsibly, with kindness and honesty. They are prepared to serve all people with the greatest care they are able to provide.

As a nurse to be, I believe that without physical health, people really have nothing at all. What a person believes (if he or she really believes it), should dictate lifestyle. Thus, if nurses have the belief that poor physical health equates to a low quality of life, the nurse's job or mission should be to help people attain and maintain an optimum state of health, functioning, and well-being. Helping an individual attain and maintain physical health should be the primary goal of the nurse, since physical needs must be met before spiritual, intellectual, and emotional needs can be met (Craven & Hirnle, 2009). After the individual's physical needs are met, the nurse can proceed to meet other needs.

Nurses should also view themselves as leaders. Since nurses believe that their purpose is to help people attain and maintain physical health, they should be role models of good physical health. Nurses who possess healthy lifestyles and are in good physical health are better able to lead others into that arena as well.

What guides my belief that nurses are to be kind and compassionate healers as well as role models? It is the same thing that draws men and women into the profession—God. Faith, *true* faith in God, is what drives nurses to action:

What does it profit, my brethren, if someone says he has faith but does not have works? Can faith save him? If a brother or sister is naked and destitute of daily food, and one of you says to them, 'Depart in peace, be warmed and filled,' but you do not give them the things which are needed for the body, what does it profit? Thus also faith by itself, if it does not have works, is dead. (James 2:14-17, New King James Version (NKJV))

Nursing spares people of dead faith. A good nurse is her brother's keeper. A good nurse looks out for the needs of others, not because it is mandated by government legislation, but because of God's love for all and His moral law, of which the nurse has become personally convinced. Nurses are the hands and feet of God. They are compelled by God to care for "the least of these" (Matt. 25:40, NKJV).

Since nursing is a way of life, nurses help all people they encounter, in whatever way possible. Nurses are drawn to wherever there is a need—schools, hospitals, nursing homes, clinics. They are also typically drawn to the dark places—the places of disease and the places where despair and hopelessness reside. They work among the forgotten and overlooked, which is why many nurses go into missionary work. Modern day nurses are also drawn to workplaces well-known for teamwork. Outside of the clinical setting, they go above and beyond, by running the errands for the neighbor who has a broken leg, helping a single mom feed her kids, and even footing the bill for someone who cannot afford his medication. Wherever they go, they put their faith into action.

My personal nursing philosophy is just that—personal. I

suppose it does have similar ideas of other theorists such as Jean Watson, who believes that interpersonal relationships are important in helping the patient heal (Johnson & Webber, 2010). I also believe that an understanding of Maslow's hierarchy of human needs is necessary for effective nursing practice (Persky, Nelson, Watson & Bent, 2008); however, I would like to say that I base my philosophy off of the ultimate standard—the Word of God.

Professional Outlook

As an employee of a nursing home, I am quick to say that a shortage of nurses is the greatest challenge to the profession of nursing today. With a lack of nurses able to provide care, those who do are unable to provide the safest and highest quality of care due to the demands of time and energy. The rising rate of obesity among young people in America poses a challenge to nursing down the road. Nurses must possess knowledge of the many diseases linked to obesity as well as all of the ways to treat the complications caused by it and how to educate clients about it. Also, a growing world population is sure to challenge nurses in the future if the nursing shortage is not resolved.

Educational Goals

Life-long learning is essential in nursing practice. Nursing, just like medicine, is an ever changing field. Nurses' knowledge and practice must be up-to-date on new flu vaccines, new treatments, and new technology in order to continue providing the best patient care.

After earning my BSN, I plan to learn as much as possible as a nurse in the working world through hands-on experience. I would also like to be highly knowledgeable, which means somewhere down the road I will be pursuing a DNP degree.

As a nurse, I desire to be the absolute best I can be in my field of work. My ultimate goal is to provide low-cost or even free care to low-income people within my community. I would like to do this via Care Vans or even open my own clinic as part of a ministry of my church. I want to build strong relationships with the people for whom I provide care. I want to be that kind, compassionate, competent nurse who leads by example and who demonstrates God's love through her actions as a nurse in practice.

Summary

The goal of nursing is to help people attain and maintain an optimal level of well-being by first meeting their physical needs.

Nurses are kind leaders driven by God's love and His word. Empathy is a new attribute that I have recently discovered in myself just since starting nursing school. I am also learning that nursing is a holistic profession, which requires a lot of knowledge in a lot of fields on the part of the nurse. This profession provides wonderful opportunity to those looking to put their faith into action.

References

American Red Cross. 2010. *History of the American Red Cross.* Retrieved from http://www.redcrosslv.org/history.html

Craven, R. F., & C. Hirnle. (2009). *Fundamentals of Nursing* (6th ed.). Philadelphia: Wolters Kluwer Health/Lippincott Williams & Wilkins.

Jonson, B. M., & P. Webber (2010). *An Introduction to Theory and Reasoning in Nursing* (3rd ed.). Philadelphia: Wolters Kluwer Health/Lippincott Williams & Wilkins.

Persky, G. J, and J. Nelson, and J. Watson, and K. Bent. (2008). Creating a Profile of a Nurse Effective in Caring. *Nursing Administration Quarterly, 32* (1), pp. 15-20.

Rebecca Parker

Philosophy of Nursing

Spring 2013

Introduction

As an individual who has lived to see the final semester in the baccalaureate nursing program, I describe myself as an inspired, driven, full-of-potential nurse-to-be with an active mind and sharpened sense of self-awareness. Throughout my journey in becoming a nurse, I have faced adversity; I have learned to let go; I have questioned my motives; I have resolved to overcome. After writing countless papers, having my hands in every possible human bodily fluid, and after witnessing the ups and downs of the human condition, I can still say that I wholeheartedly *want* to be a nurse.

The purpose of this paper is to outline my personal philosophy of nursing, including my thoughts regarding the definition and purpose of nursing, as well as assumptions and principles related to my philosophy. My beliefs and feelings about the nursing profession are the same as they were two years ago when I first developed my own philosophy of nursing. Originally, I saw the profession as one in which the nurse's goal was to help individuals attain and maintain physical health. Once this goal was achieved, the nurse could proceed to assist individuals in attaining mental, spiritual, and emotional health. I also saw the nurse as someone compelled by God to put true faith into action by caring for those in need.

Definition of Nursing

One of the reasons I chose nursing as a career is because it is a discipline that I think nicely combines many areas of study and makes them practical by applying them to real people in need. Nurses understand anatomy and physiology, chemistry, psychology, sociology, and spirituality and how they all interact to form an individual (Craven & Hirnle, 2009). The joy of nursing extends beyond the chaos of call bells, heavy work loads, tired feet, and weekend shifts; it extends beyond social services, dysfunctional families, drug addiction, and poverty. I think of nursing as caring, *genuinely* caring about the condition of one's fellow man. I think of life and its sanctity. I think of redemption and of Christ. Nursing to me is more than administering medications, assisting doctors, and setting IV pumps; it is a ministry and it is a calling.

Nursing is about helping people recover from injury or illness, usually, but not limited to physical injury or illness. Nurses are thus caregivers and nurturers. They are cheerleaders and encouragers. They are investigators, critical thinkers, and problem solvers. They are teachers. They are nightlights in the dark and friends in times of loneliness. These multiple roles of the nurse make him or her well equipped to deal with the great array of emotions and conditions that accompany the many phases of life.

When I hear the word "nursing," my mind still goes back to pictures of Clara Barton on the battlefield tending to the needs of wounded soldiers. As I think about my definition of nursing, my mind revisits how I imagined nursing as a little girl—as bandaging wounds and providing relief from pain and suffering (National Women's History Museum, 2013). This is still how I think of nursing. To me, nursing is the provision of primarily medical care, but also extends into the provision of emotional, intellectual, and spiritual care to one who is ill, wounded, disabled, or in need. It is the giving of one's self, of one's time, talents, and resources, to improve the life of another. Although some of the concepts within this definition may be similar to those of the Nursing Code of

Ethics and the American Nurses Association Standards of Professional Practice, this is my original definition of nursing (American Nurses Association [ANA], 2013).

Purpose of Nursing

The purpose of nursing, in my opinion, is to restore and improve an individual's health. This purpose is achieved by assessing the needs of people and acting to meet those needs. Restoration of health comes after a setback of some sort, whether it be from a stroke, a broken bone, or another injury. Improvement of health can also come after an injury but does not imply that an individual is sick to begin with. Generally healthy people can improve their health by eating better and exercising more, etc. This is where the nurse's role as a teacher has an impact. Nurses can teach students about the importance of time management in order to get more sleep, which does improve health; they can provide information to seniors in the community about the importance of receiving vaccines in order to prevent illness. When the purpose of nursing is fulfilled, people live healthier, fuller lives, with quality of life as a key.

I believe that the nurse is called to care, to nurture, and to relieve pain. Overall, the purpose of nursing is to heal and to improve an individual's condition. This purpose is fulfilled in a number of ways—by assessing patients' needs, by providing medication and treatment, by teaching, and sometimes simply by being present. The nurse's actions are driven by love and compassion—true love that comes only from God. Nurses are selfless and genuinely care about the wellbeing of others (ANA, 2013). The nurse has been changed by the love of God and is compelled to share this love with others. This is what drives the nurse's innate desire to heal.

Assumptions

A nurse, according to my philosophy of nursing, is one compelled by the love of God to heal and to do good. Because the nurse is consumed by the love of God and is fixed on fulfilling His purpose in the earth, the nurse is able to thrive in a culturally diverse setting. The nurse's love is God's love, and therefore does not discriminate and is not a respecter of persons (Acts 10:34, New International Version [NIV]). It knows no limits (Romans 8:38-39, NIV). Therefore, the nurse is able to provide quality care for any and every person, regardless of geographic location, the patient's skin color, gender, or background. Although cultures and languages differ, the nurse's love and compassion are fixed. Because the nurse is a detective and is able to think critically, he or she is able to efficiently assess culture and its role in the patient's life and how it affects all areas of the individual's health. The nurse, as an intelligent individual, is able to adapt the specifics of care provision in order to nurse effectively. These assumptions are consistent with those of Madeline M. Leininger's Culture Care: Diversity and Universality Theory (Johnson & Webber, 2010).

Nurses have a relationship with the communities in which they live. Because they are caring, they are active and involved in the places in which they live and take pride in their communities. They are able to apply nursing skills to a group of people in order to improve the quality of life for individuals within the community. They care for an entire population of people. At the community level, the nurse works as a collaborator, an intermediary, and as a problem solver. Interpersonal relations play a part in the nurse's role in improving the community. The nurse becomes a partner, as Peplau states in her theory of Interpersonal Relations in Nursing, with the community in order to improve it. The nurse establishes a relationship with individuals in the community in order to identify a problem, establish expectations of the nurse-patient/community relationship, and work to resolve the problem. The nurse within the community, according to Peplau, serves as a teacher, a resource, a leader, a technical expert, and a surrogate in order to fulfill the purpose of nursing (Johnson & Webber, 2010).

I believe that the professional nurse has strong relationships with many other members within the health care team. Nurses work with and alongside doctors, physician assistants, nurse practitioners, nurse aides, physical therapists, and many others as part of a team effort in healing and improving lives. Thus, nurses communicate well with other professionals in order to understand their roles and goals for the patient so that a clear plan is established. The nurse is a team player and understands her unique role and function as well as the unique roles of other health care professionals in achieving a common goal for the improvement of a patient's condition. Theorist Virginia Henderson is known for developing a definition of nursing. She believed that a clear definition of the role of the nurse would outline the functions, duties, expectations, and limitations of the professional nurse. By having a clear definition of nursing, the nurse and her role is distinct from that of other members of the health care team. This enables the nurse to work effectively so that her purpose is fulfilled and the patient's life is improved (Johnson & Webber, 2010).

Principles of Professional Practice

As stated earlier, I believe that the nurse is filled with God's love and is driven by it to care for people. For this reason, the two principles that I apply to my professional practice are commands from God Himself found in the Bible. The first is "Owe nothing to anyone—except your obligation to love one another. If you love your neighbor, you fulfill the requirements of God's law" (Romans 13:8, New Living Translation). The other is well known as the Golden Rule : "Do to others as you would have them do to you" (Luke 6:27, NIV). In this same passage, Jesus talks about loving one's enemies, giving without expecting anything in return, and about being merciful, especially to those who seem undeserving. These are all principles that I believe the nurse is to practice and live by.

Throughout my clinical experiences in the nursing program, I have on many occasions applied these rules. As a nursing student, before even entering the hospital each clinical rotation, I review exactly what is expected of me as a student nurse. When in the hospital, I am careful to make sure that I fulfill the requirements that are expected of me. I am mindful to give of myself, to hold nothing back that is within my capacity to give. In this way, I am not in debt to those I care for and to those who have allowed me into the hospital. Specifically, I loved a psychiatric patient simply by listening to her share her story. I loved her by offering to pray for her as well as by encouraging her to continue fighting her battles. I Corinthians 13:4 describes love as patient and kind. I loved this depressed woman in her darkest hours by simply being a listening ear and a soft, sweet voice of hope.

    I applied the Golden Rule during my rotation in the Labor and Delivery unit. There was a young mom who, after delivering her baby, said she was hungry. As someone who hates to hunger myself, and after realizing that she had not eaten during her long labor, I realized that she must really have been starving. When she showed disinterest for the food on the tray, I took the initiative to ask her exactly what she would like to eat. When she requested a cheeseburger, French fries, and a cold lemonade, I made a special trip to the cafeteria and came back to hand-deliver her exact request. This is something I would like to have done for me, so I did it for her. Thus, the Golden Rule was fulfilled.

Conclusion

Nurses are a unique group of people. They are smart, compassionate, and kind. They assess, identify needs, and work tirelessly to meet those needs. They are versatile, able to handle all kinds of situations and people. They are fueled not by a paycheck or by self-gratification, but rather by the limitless love of God. Nursing is the provision of care to provide physical, intellectual, spiritual, and emotional restoration and improvement. It is healing. Nurses are involved in the community and work well with other members of the health care team. They adhere to a high moral code, written by God.

My personal philosophy has not changed from two years ago when I first developed it; however, revisiting it has reawakened my desire to be a nurse and put it into practice. My personal philosophy of nursing drives me to be the best nurse I can be, to give my life for something greater than myself, and to restore and improve the lives of those for whom I care.

References

American Nurses Association. (2013). *Nursing Principles*. Retrieved from

http://www.nursingworld.org/MainMenuCategories/ThePracticeofProfessionalNursing/NursingStandards/ANAPrinciples

Craven, R. F. & Hirnle, C.J. (2009). *Fundamentals of nursing: human health and function.* (6h ed.). Philadelphia, PA: Wolters Kluwer Health/Lippincott Williams & Wilkins.

Johnson, B.M. & Webber, P.B. (2010). *An introduction to theory and reasoning in nursing* (3rd ed.). Philadelphia, PA: Wolters Kluwer Health/Lippincott Williams & Wilkins.

National Women's History Museum. (2013). *Clara Barton 1821-1912*. Retrieved from http://www.nwhm.org/education-resources/biography/biographies/clara-barton/

Cultural Reflection Paper: The Culture of the Elderly and the Culture of Obesity

Fall 2011

One patient I took care of during the med-surge clinical this semester was a 76-year-old female. She was a 5'4, 170 pound post-operative patient recovering from a total left knee replacement. Her medical history included chronic knee pain as a result of osteoarthritis, asthma, pre-diabetes, high blood pressure, reflux, and hypothyroidism. This patient's older age places her in the category of an elderly client. Her body mass index (BMI) of 30.9 indicates that she is obese (Ignatavicius & Workman, 2011).

Both old age and obesity are two common themes in the current health care system. Elderly persons, those considered 65 years old or older, make up a culture of their own. In 2007, there were 37.9 million elderly people living in the United States. People over the age of 65 are the most frequent users of health care services. The most common health problems of this population are 1) arthritis, 2) hypertension, and 3) heart disease. Depression and diabetes mellitus are also very common. A limited income due to retirement and an inability to work are other characteristics of the culture of the elderly (Meiner, 2011). Many older people live alone, and are therefore the ones responsible for their own care, which can be challenging when issues of transportation and navigating the health care system are faced (Horton & Johnson, 2010).

The culture of obesity has a significant effect on the United States' health care system. Currently, an estimated 32% of Americans over the age of 20 are obese (meaning the individual has a BMI of 30 or greater). The obese patient faces numerous additional health problems compared to a patient of normal weight. Obese patients are at greater risk for contracting diabetes mellitus, hypertension, and osteoarthritis. Many of these preventable diseases contribute to the increased cost of health care. Obesity is the second leading cause of preventable death in the United States (Ignatavicius & Workman, 2011). The culture of obesity cannot be properly discussed without mention of nutrition and exercise, which often requires a look into lifestyle and home life. Although the obese patient presents numerous challenges to providing care, the registered nurse possesses the necessary knowledge and skill needed to combat the culture of obesity (Drake et al., 2008).

As a member of the elderly culture, my patient faces significant challenges. Age is likely the main culprit for her osteoarthritis. It is also not uncommon for high blood pressure to accompany older age (Ignatavicius & Workman, 2011). My patient lives alone, which has the potential to create anxiety when seeking medical care. I noticed that she relied on her daughter for help. She used her cell phone to ask her daughter to bring a medication to the hospital. I believe the patient will depend on her daughter for transportation during the post-operative phase. Lack of transportation is a major barrier to accessing health care for the elderly population (Horton & Johnson, 2010).

Living alone also has the potential to create feelings of isolation among older people. Isolation can frequently come from within the health care system as well. One study found that elderly people feel the most common barrier to their seeking health care is a lack of responsiveness from doctors about their concerns (Horton & Johnson, 2010). I noticed that my patient asked me numerous questions concerning her care. She asked me when her stitches would be removed as well as the uses for her medications. This does not necessarily mean that her questions, if previously asked, were not addressed, but it is a possibility.

Ageism, "a deep-seated uneasiness on the part of young and middle-aged—a personal revulsion and distaste for growing old, disease, disability; and fear of powerlessness, 'uselessness', and death," (Meiner, 2011, p.10) has a great impact on health care for those in the elderly culture. Many health care workers still believe, despite research showing the contrary, that high blood pressure is a normal part of aging. This attitude can keep the elderly from getting proper screening, taking preventative measures, and from receiving treatment. The belief that many health ailments are normal with aging can have a huge impact on care. One study at Johns Hopkins Medical School found that 80% of medical students would aggressively treat pneumonia in a child, but only 56% would do the same for an elderly patient (Currey, 2008).

All of these issues, from the health complications of old age to the negative repercussions of ageism, affect nursing care. Since the elderly population is the fastest growing segment of the population and since many older nurses are now seeking retirement, more nurses are needed to provide care (Meiner, 2011). Since those living in the elderly culture are often faced with the barriers of limited income, lack of social support, and no transportation, they are less likely to seek medical care and obtain basic recommended preventative screenings. Nursing care needs to focus on reaching this segment of the population (Horton & Johnson, 2011). Physical assessments must be thorough for older clients, as they often have several chronic conditions (Meiner, 2011). Nurses are in a perfect position to establish trusting relationships with these clients. Nurses can refer them to the proper social services and take the time to answer their questions (Horton & Johnson, 2011).

The culture of obesity is well-noted within the health care system. My patient chose to have a knee replacement because of osteoarthritis that was exacerbated by her excess weight. Her high blood pressure and pre-diabetes were also likely related to her obesity. The co-morbidities associated with obesity create additional costs for obtaining treatment (Drake et al., 2008).

In a study done by Drake et al. (2008), special equipment needs were found to be the most common barrier to providing care to morbidly obese patients. Inadequate staffing needed to provide care to the morbidly obese was also seen as a hindrance to care (Drake et al., 2008). Just as elderly patients face ageism (Meiner,

2011), obese patients come against stereotypes when seeking health care. Negative nurse attitudes regarding overweight patients, such as viewing them as gluttons or sloths responsible for their obesity, can contribute to poor nursing care and even no nursing care for these patients (Drake et al., 2008).

The rising rate of obesity in the U.S. has significant implications for nursing practice. Special equipment, such as larger blood pressure cuffs and transferring equipment, needs to be accessible to nursing staff. Adequate staffing should be a priority for the nurse manager. Meeting both of these conditions will promote safety for both nurses and obese patients and will improve quality of care. Nurses must examine their own attitudes concerning obesity. By having the right attitude, they can encourage obese patients to do all they can to control their weight and attain a healthy lifestyle. Nurses are in the perfect spot to provide patient education to reduce the incidence of obesity in society and to treat the existing complications of the disease (Drake et al., 2008).

The culture of the elderly and the culture of obesity are both commonly encountered within the health care system. Members of these cultures have special needs and face numerous challenges to receiving adequate care. The elderly fight the challenges of living alone, lack of transportation, lack of resources, and ageism (Horton & Johnson, 2010). The obese patient faces many health complications and stereotypes from caregivers (Drake et al., 2008). Nurses must extend compassion to these two groups and overcome the issue of prejudice (Horton & Johnson, 2010; Drake et al., 2008). The concept of culture within the health care setting must not be neglected, as it certainly has an impact on the care that patients receive.

References

Currey, Richard. (2008). Ageism in health care: time for a change. *Aging Well, 1*(1), 16. Retrieved from http://www.agingwellmag.com/archive/winter08p16.shtml

Drake, D.J., Baker, G., Engelke, M.K., McAuliffe, M., Pokomy, M., Swanson, M., . . . Rose, M.A. (2008). Challenges in caring for the morbidly obese: differences by practice setting. *Southern Online Journal of Nursing Research, 8*(6).

Horton, S. & Johnson, R.J. (2010). Improving access to health care for uninsured elderly patients. *Public Health Nursing, 27*(4), 362-370. doi: 10.1111/j.1525-1446.2010.00866.x

Ignatavicius, D.D. & Workman, L.M. (2011). *Medical-surgical nursing: patient-centered collaborative care.* (6th ed.). St. Louis, MO: Mosby.

Meiner, S.E. *Gerontologic nursing.* (2011). (4th ed.). St. Louis, MO: Mosby.

School of Nursing

Pre-Clinical Form

Patient Information Sheet

Student Name <u>Rebecca</u> Date of Experience <u>1/28/11</u>

Patient Initials (N341 primary or secondary patient) <u>Code Status</u> /Advanced Directive? <u>Full Code</u>   DOB:

Patient's Age <u>70</u> Sex <u>M</u> Race <u>African American</u> Marital Status <u>W</u>

Religious Pref. _____ Occupation

Allergies _____

Smokes <u>has never smoked, has never used smokeless tobacco</u>

ETOH <u>not found in chart</u>   Adm. Date <u>1/28/11</u> Fall Risk? <u>Yes</u>

Primary Caregiver/Support System <u>self???</u>

History of Present Illness

Pt was admitted to ED via Public Rescue. When EMS arrived, he was unresponsive. AED delivered one shock; CPR was administered. He also had agonal breathing and a weak pulse at time of EMS arrival. He presented to ED with cardiac arrest and was subsequently found to be hypokalemic. In the ED he was given NS 125cc/hr IV and KCl 10mEq IV. Cardiac arrest appears to be a first-time problem for the pt. Problem was resolved in ER. Pt has had previous ER visits, 6 last month for various problems, including AMS, back pain, ankle injury; dialysis shunt problem; vascular access problem; fecal impaction; fall.

Past Medical History: PVD, anemia, reflux, C-diff, MI, DVT (LLE with IVC filter on chronic anticoagulation), CHF (unspecified), CAD (with stent), HTN (controlled with meds), hypercalcemia, hyperkalemia, DM (BG was 198 in ED), elevated cholesterol, BPH, renal disorder (dialysis M/W/F), kidney disease, ulcer, arthropathy (unspecified), hip fracture (left), muscle atrophy, unspecified epilepsy without mention of intractable epilepsy, headache, leg cramps, stroke (on CT, no clinical history), ESRD (does void), refusal of blood transfusions since he is a Jehovah's witness, hemodialysis (M/W/F), sickle cell anemia (trait), reduced hearing bilaterally.

Primary Medical Diagnosis

Cardiac Arrest, not to be mistaken with heart attack, is the sudden stopping of all heart function. It occurs when the heart's electrical conduction system stops working because of the presence of arrhythmias (the most common being ventricular fibrillation). It can occur in people who have no diagnosis of heart disease and it occurs abruptly or shortly after symptoms occur. The major warning sign of cardiac arrest is sudden unresponsiveness in a person. A person experiencing cardiac arrest does not respond to voice or to touch. A person experiencing cardiac arrest will die within minutes unless CPR and/or defibrillation (a "shock") is provided. Risk factors for this condition include previous MI, arrhythmias, use of cardiac medications, blood vessel abnormalities, and a thickened heart muscle. Emergency treatment consists of CPR and AED use. Long-term treatment typically requires identification of the cause and management of risk factors ("Cardiac Arrest," 2011).

Secondary Medical Diagnoses

Hypokalemia is the term used to define a low potassium level, and is indicated by a blood serum potassium level of less than 3.5 mEq/L. Potassium is the major cation of the intracellular fluid. It functions in depolarization and generation of action potentials and regulates protein synthesis and glucose use as well as heart and skeletal muscle contractions. Common causes include inappropriate or excessive use of diuretics, digitalis, or corticosteroids; increased secretion of aldosterone, Cushing's syndrome, diarrhea, vomiting, wound drainage, prolonged nasogastric suction, heat-induced excessive sweating, renal disease, and NPO status. Signs and symptoms of hypokalemia include reduced responsiveness of nerve and muscle cells to stimuli; skeletal muscle weakness; shallow respirations; flaccid paralysis (in extreme cases); thready and weak pulse; dysrhythmia; orthostatic hypotension; AMS evidenced by irritability, anxiety, lethargy, and confusion; decreased peristalsis and hypoactive bowel sounds; abdominal distention; nausea, and paralytic ileus (in severe cases). Treatment consists of administration of potassium chloride potassium gluconate, potassium citrate supplements, or potassium-sparing diuretics; safety measures; and respiratory monitoring (Ignatavicius & Workman, 2011).

Surgical Procedures (if applicable)

March 2006 ORIF upper/lower ext (non-hip) post proc osset hip fx

2008 Ivc filter placement

date not specified Chg-stent coronary other

date unknown leg surgery-left leg chronically larger than right

date unknown hx dialysis catheter

date unknown hx dialysis fistula or graft

3/23/2006 A/v fistula Kauffman

3/23/2006 hx vascular surgery-left arm brachiocephalic with AV fistula, good artery, good vein, good thrill

10/16/06 hx vascular surgery-ligate left AV fistula and create left 1st stage basilica vein transposition. The vein appeared adequate, the artery good.

1/11/10 hx vascular surgery-exploration left basilica vein and left upper arm bucket handle type avg with 6 mm ptfe

6/2010 - hx vascular surgery-AV accessx2 separate sheaths, AVF-gram with venous runoff, first order central catheter and selective SVC-gram, 10 mm left innominate balloon angioplasty, retrograde brachial angiogram

Patient Education: Include what you would teach the patient/and or family even if you do not anticipate actually being able to provide the teaching (attach a sheet if necessary)

This pt will likely need education concerning diabetes mellitus. He will most likely need to be taught how to check his own blood sugar level at home. He will need to be taught how to give an insulin injection. I would like to teach him about the importance of exercise and a healthy diet, as these interventions will help improve his cardiovascular status as well. His exercise must not be strenuous due to his cardiac issues. He will benefit from a low sodium, low-fat diet that is rich in fruits and vegetables. He will also need education about his medication regimen before he is discharged. Also, I plan to teach him about heart disease and its complications, such as the symptoms of an impending heart attack (arm pain, chest pain)/cardiac arrest (unresponsiveness) and when and how to seek help.

Discharge Planning: **Yes! We think about discharge even on the day of admission! This is a critical thinking exercise. There is no wrong answer.**

- Do you think this patient will be able to go to their previous living situation?
- What anticipated resources will the patient need to care for self at home?
- What activities should be planned prior to discharge to

prepare the patient for home care?

This patient has numerous chronic conditions that require medical management. Depending on his level of competency and ability to care for himself, he should be able to return home. He will need a way to check his blood sugar at home as well as equipment to manage his diabetes (insulin, syringes, etc.). He will also need devices to assist him with mobility, such as a wheelchair or walker since he does have a cast on his foot. He might need oxygen at home as well. He could benefit from nutritional counseling as well as physical therapy to help him improve his mobility.

Recent Pertinent Diagnostic Procedures *and* Results: (X-rays, scans, EKG's, ultrasounds. etc, include the dates)

2/18 ECG- Pt has IVCD. EF is 36% with wall motion abnormality. Mildly increased left ventricular cavity size. Mild mitral regurgitation.

2/21 PICC LINE-PICC line stable and in place in R arm.

2/22 CAT Scan-CAT Scan of Abdomen/Pelvis shows

intraparenchymal hemorrhage within the left psoas muscle; severe distention of the colon with an air-fluid level within the sigmoid colon with distention measuring 15.1 cm in diameter; increased perinephric stranding particularly around the right kidney may represent pyelonephritis. Cardiomegaly is present. Dependent atelectasis is present with bilateral small pleural effusions suggested.

2/25 X-Ray- Abdominal X-Ray shows gas filled transverse and distal colon; gas dilation of sigmoid colon. An IVC filter is noted and appears stable. Atherosclerosis and left femoral hardware noted.

Oxygen therapy: No.

Pulse Oximetry: Yes.

Diet orders: Mechanical soft

Accucheck: yes; at 0600 and before & after meals

IV Fluids and rate: PICC in R arm

Activity orders: ???

Vital Sign frequency: q 4 h

Treatments: (NG tube, chest tube, dressing change): Pt has a PICC

Lab Tests	Normal Values	Results/ Date	Results/ Date	Results/ Date	Rationale for abnormal values
RBC	4.20-5.30	2.44 *	2.37 *	2.79 *	anemia, kidney disease, dietary deficiency
WBC	4.6-13.2	8.5	6.9	7.3	
HGB	12.0-16.0	5.8 *	5.6 *	6.6 *	anemia, renal disease, dietary deficiency
HCT	35.0-45.0%	18.7 *	18.3 *	21.9 *	anemia, renal disease, dietary deficiency
Platelets	135-420	419	397	385	
NA	136-145 mmol/L	142	---	---	
K	3.5-5.5 mmol/L	---	3.6 on 2/26	3.6	
CL	100-108 mmol/L	103	---	---	
CO2	21-32 mmol/L	22	---	---	
Glucose	74-99 mg/dL	178 *	---	---	DM
BUN	1-18 mg/dL	45 *	---	---	kidney disease
Creatinine	0.6-1.3 mg/dL (for adult males); 0.5-1.1 for adult females)	7.1 *	---	---	kidney disease
Albumin	3.5-5 mg/dL	3.2 * on 2/13, 3.3 on 2/19	---	---	kidney disease

THE TRUTH ABOUT NURSING

PT	11.0-12.5 sec.	17.0 *	14.0 *		Vitamin K deficiency (hypokalemia)
PTT	30-40 sec.	not in chart	---	---	
INR	0.8-1.1	1.69 *	1.37 * (1.33 * on 2/26)		Vitamin K deficiency (hypokalemia)
Blood Culture 2/25	negative	no growth	---	---	
Wound Culture (site)	normal/negative	abnormal- gram- negative rod (lactose ferment 9000 org/mL * on 2/25			Pt has an infection.
C-Diff 2/25	negative	negative	---	---	
Drug Levels	---	---			
Urinalysis 2/25					
urine protein	0-8 mg/dL; 50-80/ 24 hrs (at rest); <250 mg/24 hr (during exercise)	>= 300 *	---	---	kidney disease
urine glucose	negative	negative	---	---	
urine occult blood	none	moderate *	---	---	kidney disease, infection, meds???
urine nitrite	None	positive *	---	---	possible UTI
urine leukocyte	Negative	moderate *	---	---	bacterial infection in urinary tract
WBC urine	Negative	packed *	---	---	possible UTI
RBC urine	negative	many *	---	---	possible UTI

List all STANDING and PRN medications and rationale for why this patient is receiving these meds.

Acetaminophen (Tylenol): Mechanism of Action (MOA):

Appears to inhibit prostaglandin synthesis in the CNS and to a lesser extent, blocks pain impulses through peripheral action. Acts centrally on hypothalamic heat-regulating center, produces vasodilation. Results in antipyresis; produces analgesic effect. Dosing: 650 mg oral q 4 h PRN. Adverse Effects: Watch for hypersensitivity reaction (rash, fever). Nursing Considerations: Do not exceed 4000 mg per day. Give without regard to meals. Tablets may be crushed. Interacts with alcohol (long-term use), hepatotoxic meds, warfarin (may cause increased risk for bleeding). Monitor temperature.

albuterol (Proventil) solution 2.5 mg: MOA: bronchodilator (adrenergic agonist) – Stimulates beta2-adrenergic receptors in the lungs, resulting in relaxation of bronchial smooth muscles. Alleviates bronchospasm and reduces resistance of airways. Dosing: 2.5 mg inhalation q 4 h PRN respiratory. Adverse Effects: May cause dry, irritated mouth or throat. May cause headache. Too much stimulation can cause palpitations, extrasystole (extra or skipped beats), tachycardia, and angina pectoris, elevated B/P. Beta-blockers antagonize this drug. May increase risk of arrhythmias when taken with digoxin. Thyroid hormones enhance risk of coronary insufficiency in pts with CAD. MAOIs and TCAs increase risk of cardiovascular effects. May increase blood glucose level; may decrease serum K+. Offer emotional support to the patient with anxiety (due to difficulty breathing). Monitor depth, rate, and rhythm of respirations. Asses lung sounds for rales and wheezes. Teach patient to not take more than 2 inhalations at one time, to increase fluid intake, to rinse the mouth with water immediately after inhalation, and to avoid excessive caffeine.

artificial tear (LACRILUBE S.O.P.) ophthalmic ointment 1 Application: MOA: lubricant; artificial tear ointment. Dosing: 1 application to both eyes q 12 h. Adverse Effects: A side effect is blurred vision (should go away). Redness, irritation, changes in vision are also possible side effects. Watch for signs of allergic reaction (itching, hives, rash, fever, etc.). . Nursing Considerations: Apply 0.25 inches to inside of each eyelid. Pull lower eyelid away from eye to make a pouch. Squeeze a thin strip of ointment into the pouch without touching the eye. Have pt close eye for 1-2 minutes.

carvedilol (Coreg) tablet 6.25 mg: MOA: "beta-adrenergic blocker; antihypertensive – possesses nonselective beta-blocking and alpha-adrenergic-blocking activity. Causes vasodilation.

Reduces CO, exercise-induced tachycardia, reflex orthostatic tachycardia; reduces PVR" (Hodgson & Kozior, 2011). Dose: 6.25 mg oral daily with meals. Adverse Effects: CCBs increase risk of cardiac conduction disturbances. Diuretics and other antihypertensives may potentiate hypotensive effects. Cimetidine may increase concentrations. May increase concentration of cyclosporine, digoxin. May decrease effect of insulin, oral hypoglycemic. Rifampin decreases concentration. May increase bilirubin, transaminases, serum creatinine, PT. Frequent yet mild side effects include fatigue and dizziness. Diarrhea, back pain, rhinitis, and bradycardia are also less common SEs. Hypoglycemia may occur in diabetic pts with previously controlled DM. Nursing Considerations: Assess B/P and apical pulse immediately before administering this drug. Hold and contact physician if pulse is 60 or less or if systolic BP is less than 90 mmHg. Monitor BP for hypotension and respirations for dyspnea. Assess pulse for quality, rate, rhythm. Monitor I &O and assess for signs of CHF (JVD, peripheral edema, night cough, dyspnea). Tell pt that Coreg takes 1-2 weeks to have full antihypertensive effect, to not abruptly stop taking this med, and to monitor salt and alcohol intake.

ciprofloxacin (CIPRO) 400 mg/200 mL IVPB 400 mg: MOA: fluoroquinolone; anti-infective – inhibits enzyme, DNA gyrase in susceptible bacteria, interferes with bacterial cell replication. Kills bacteria. Dosing: 400 mg IV q24 h. Adverse Effects: Antacids, iron preparations, sucralfate may decrease absorption. May increase effects of caffeine, oral anticoagulants. May decrease concentration of phenytoin. May cause theophylline toxicity. Frequent side effects include nausea, diarrhea, dyspepsia, vomiting, constipation, flatulence, confusion, crystalluria. Adverse effects include superinfection, nephropathy, cardiopulmonary arrest, allergic reaction. Incompatible with "calcium gluconate, diltiazem dobutamine, dopamine, lidocaine, lipids, lorazepam, magnesium, Versed, and KCl" (Lilley et al., 2011). Nursing Considerations: Assess pt's hx of hypersensitivity to ciprofloxacin, quinolones. Monitor bowel activity. Encourage pt to drink plenty of fluids. Monitor for dizziness, headache, visual changes, tremors. Assess for joint and chest pain. Obtain urinalysis; observe for crystalluria prior to and during treatment. Encourage pt to ingest plenty of ascorbic acid (from cranberry juice, citrus fruit) to reduce risk for crystalluria and to avoid antacids.

epoetin alfa (non-oncology) (EPOGEN;PROCRIT) injection 20,000 units. MOA: erythropoietin – stimulates division and differentiation of erythroid progenitor cells in bone marrow. Induces red blood cell formation, releases reticulocytes from bone marrow. Dosing: 20,000 sub-q given during every dialysis. Adverse Effects: * Black box warning – increased risk of serious cardiovascular events, thromboembolic events. An increase in RBC volume can enhance blood clotting. Heparin and iron supplement dosages may need to be adjusted. May increase BUN, serum phosphorus, K, creatinine, uric acid, Na+. May decrease bleeding time, iron concentration, and serum ferritin. Frequent side effects of this drug for pts with chronic renal failure are hypertension, headache, nausea, and arthralgia. Adverse effects include hypertensive encephalopathy, thrombosis, CVA, MI, and seizures. Nursing Considerations: Assess BP before administering this drug. Consider that pt needs supplemental iron therapy. Serum iron should be >20%. Establish baseline CBC. Monitor Hct level (if it increases >4 pts in 2 wks, dosage should be reduced). Monitor BUN, serum uric acid, creatinine, phosphorus, potassium. Teach pt to inform physician if severe headache develops and to avoid potentially hazardous activities for first 90 days (d/t risk of seizures).

famotidine (PEPCID) injection 20 mg. MOA: H2 receptor antagonist; antiulcer – gastric acid secretion inhibitor. Inhibits histamine action H2 receptors of parietal cells. Inhibits gastric acid secretion. Dosing: 20 mg IV push daily (2 mL = 20 mg of 10mg/mL. Adverse Effects: May decrease absorption of itraconazole, ketoconazole. May increase hepatic enzymes. (IV) incompatibility with amphotericin B complex, Maxipime, Rocephin, Lasix, and Zosyn. Headache is an occasional side effect. Nursing Considerations: Dilute in 5-10 mL of normal saline and administer over 1-2 minutes. Monitor daily stool pattern. Monitor for diarrhea, constipation, headache. May be taken without regard to meals. Teach pt to avoid large amounts of caffeine and aspirin.

Insulin 7030 (NOVOLIN/HUMULIN) 100 units/mL (70-30) injection 16 units. MOA: antidiabetic – facilitates passage of glucose, K+, Mg+ across cellular membranes of skeletal and cardiac muscle and adipose tissue. Promotes conversion of glucose to glycogen in the liver. Controls glucose levels in diabetic pts. This is a fixed-combination of insulin consisting of 70% NPH (an intermediate-acting insulin with onset of 1-2 hours and duration of 16-24 hrs+) and 30% regular human insulin (a rapid-acting insulin with onset of 10-30 minutes and duration of action of 3-5 hours). Most common SE is hypoglycemia. Localized redness is also a side effect. Give 30 minutes AC per medical staff policy.

insulin lispro (HUMALOG vial) injection 1-10 units: MOA: rapid-acting insulin, exogenous insulin, antidiabetic – facilitates passage of glucose, K+, Mg+ across cellular membranes of skeletal and cardiac muscle and adipose tissue. Promotes conversion of glucose to glycogen in the liver. Controls glucose levels in diabetic pts. Dosing: 1-10 units sub-q injection 4 times daily after meals & at bedtime. Adverse Effects: Most common SE is hypoglycemia. Localized redness is also a side effect. Nursing considerations: Check blood sugar before administration. Onset is within 15-30 minutes; be sure food is readily available. Assess for hypoglycemia (cool, wet skin, tremors, dizziness, headache, anxiety, tachycardia). Teach pt about diet and exercise.

sodium chloride (NORMAL SALINE) 0.9% infusion and albumin, human 25% injection: MOA: * isotonic fluid –

decreases colloid osmotic pressure. plasma protein fraction; blood derivative – blood volume expander, reduces hemoconcentration and blood viscosity. Dosing: 500 mL IV PRN. If systolic blood pressure <100 mmHg, give to achieve SBP at 100 mmHG 25 g IV PRN. (100 mL = 25 g of 25 g/100 mL). If systolic blood pressure <100 mmHg, give to achieve SBP at 100 mmHG. Do not exceed 1 mL/min in pts with normal plasma volume; 2-3 mL/min in pts with hypoproteinemia. Adverse Effects: Monitor for fluid overload. Albumin: No significant drug interactions. May increase serum alkaline phosphatase concentration. IV incompatible with lipids, Versed, Vancomycin (* note: pt is on this), and Isoptin. Occasional side effect is hypotension. Fluid overload may occur, indicated by increased BP, JVD, pulmonary edema. Nursing Considerations: Monitor IV site for phlebitis, infiltration.

Obtain baseline BP, pulse, respirations before administering. Assess for fluid overload. Monitor I & O. Check for skin flushing.

Concept Map for Pt

# 1 Decreased Cardiac Output r/t decreased oxygenation, alteration in heart conduction, cardiac muscle disease	# 2 Impaired Gas Exchange r/t altered oxygen supply, altered oxygen-carrying capacity of blood	# 3 Ineffective Tissue Perfusion r/t impaired transport of oxygen, interruption in blood flow, decreased hemoglobin concentration in blood, altered affinity of hemoglobin for oxygen.
mitral valve regurgitation	confusion, AMS hypoxia, atelectasis, anemia, ESRD, CHF	weak peripheral pulses, AMS, dysrhythmias
EF 39 %		
atherosclerosis	Hgb 6.6, Hct 21.9	BUN 45, creatinine 7.1
cardiomegaly	procrit	Hgb 6.6, Hct 21.9
cardiac arrest, MI, PVD, DVT, CHF, CAD, HTN	iron sucrose ipratroprium albuterol	MI, CHF, anemia, PVD, CAD, HTN, ESRD
Coreg	Elevate HOB, provide O2 per physician's order, provide environment conducive to rest, organize nursing care	Elevate HOB, provide O2 per physician's order, provide environment conducive to rest, organize nursing care.
hydralazine		
Maintain optimal fluid balance.		
Maintain hemodynamic parameters at prescribed levels (human albumin)	Assess respirations, noting quality, rate, rhythm, depth, and breathing effort. Assess for tachycardia, restlessness, irritability, limited diaphragm excursion.	Assess capillary refill, edema, hypovolemia, compartment syndrome.
Maintain physical and emotional rest: restrict activity, provide quiet environment, organize nursing and medical care.		Assist with slow position changes.
		Place pt in semi-to high-Fowler's position as tolerated.
		Administer O2 therapy as prescribed.

#4 Risk for Infection r/t malnutrition, IV devices, chronic disease	70 YO AA M Cardiac Arrest, hypokalemia	#5 Risk for Falls r/t history of fall, old age, hearing difficulties, polypharmacy, unfamiliar environment.
PICC line	Past Medical hx: PVD, anemia, reflux, C-diff, MI, DVT, CHF (unspecified), CAD, HTN, hypercalcemia, hyperkalemia, DM (BG was 190 in ED), elevated cholesterol, BPH, ulcer, arthropathy, muscle atrophy, unspecified epilepsy, stroke, ESRD, sickle cell anemia.	age 72
fecal management system		reduced hearing in L ear
Foley catheter		Answer call lights immediately.
Compromised immune system r/t age		Avoid use of restraints to reduce falls.
Lengthy hospital stay		Ensure appropriate lighting in room.
antibiotic therapy (risk for superinfection)		Use side rails on bed as needed.
current and previous infections. Monitor for redness, swelling, increased pain, purulent drainage, elevated temperature, appearance of urine. Assess nutritional status, including weight. Wash hands thoroughly.		Place all important items within patient's reach.
		Move pt to room near nurse's station (Gulanik & Myers, 2011).
Encourage intake of protein and calorie-rich foods. Encourage coughing and deep breathing.		

References

Cardiac Arrest. (2011). American Heart Association. Retrieved from

http://www.heart.org/HEARTORG/Conditions/More/Cardiac

Arrest/Long-Term-

Treatment-for-Cardiac-Arrest_UCM_307916_Article.jsp

Info from concept map: Gulanick, M. & Myers, J.L. (2011).

Nursing care plans: diagnoses,

interventions, and outcomes. St.Louis, MO: Elsevier.

Source of all meds (unless otherwise noted):

Hodgson, B.B. & Kozior, R.J. (2011). *Saunders Nursing Drug*

Handbook. St.Louis: Elsevier.

Ignatavicius, D.D. & Workman, M.L. (2011*). Medical-surgical*

nursing:

patient-centered collaborative care. (6th ed). St.Louis: Mosby.

Lacrilube. (2011). Walgreens. Retrieved from

http://www.walgreens.com/marketing/library/finddrug/druginf

o1.html;jsessionid=Rkqx

24qLORUy80FSxkksvA**.p_dotcom63?particularDrug=L

acri-Lube&id=2881

* Lilley, L.L., Collins, S.R., Harrington, S., & Snyder, J.S. (2011).

Pharmacology and the

nursing process. (6th ed.). St.Louis: Elsevier

Nephrocaps. (2012). Drugs.com. Retrieved from http://www.drugs.com/cdi/nephrocaps.html

Client Case Study

Fall 2012

Submitted in partial fulfillment of the requirements in the course

Clinical Management of Adults III

Client Case Study

The purpose of this paper is to present a patient cared for during the Critical Care rotation this semester. Both the original and revised concept maps used to plan care for this client will be expanded upon and information from the humanities, sciences, and research will be presented to provide a thorough discussion of the patient. Both medical and nursing diagnoses will be explained as well as appropriate nursing interventions and outcomes. An evaluation of the patient's progress will also be discussed. Research will be presented to support nursing care.

This paper will explore the case of a 55-year-old African American female patient with a history of type II diabetes mellitus, cerebrovascular accident, hypertension, hypercholesterolemia, bipolar disorder, depression, and anxiety. She was cared for over four different days in two separate weeks during this rotation at the Regional Medical Center (RMC). The first week in which she was cared for was when she was admitted to the intensive care unit (ICU) with the diagnoses of altered mental status, dehydration, acute renal failure, and acute pancreatitis. She was discharged from the hospital after receiving care for these conditions but was readmitted two days later for altered mental status and fever, for which she was found to be septic. Acute sepsis will be the focus of this discussion, as it was the reason for her most recent admission to the ICU.

Medical Diagnosis

Sepsis is a term used to describe the body's response to an invading microorganism. When a foreign agent, whether it is bacteria, fungi, or virus, etc., enters the body, the immune system reacts to protect the host. Neutrophils, macrophages, and other cells of the host's immune system are activated. The patient will often exhibit an elevated white blood cell (WBC) count, defined as a count greater than 12,000 cells/mm3 or a very low WBC count (less than 4,000 cells/mm3). The release of cytokines and other chemical mediators in the body causes widespread inflammation and damage to the lining of blood vessels. There is increased permeability of capillaries (small blood vessels), which causes fluid to leak into intravascular space and create massive vasodilation. Blood pressure drops. Damaged blood vessels result in decreased perfusion to vital organs in the body. This results in organ dysfunction and can lead to death (Urden, Stacy, & Lough, 2010).

The clinical manifestations of sepsis include hypotension, evidenced by a systolic blood pressure (SBP) of less than 90 mmHg; serum lactate of greater than 1; temperature greater than 98.6 degrees F; a heart rate of greater than 90; and a respiratory rate greater than 20/min (Urden, Stacy, & Lough, 2010). This patient had a temperature of 106 degrees Fahrenheit when she was readmitted to the emergency department. She also had a lactic acid of 2.9 and a WBC count of 4.0. An organism was never identified as the cause of the sepsis, as her blood and urine cultures and chest x-ray were all negative. During this patient's second admission to the ICU (for sepsis), hypotension was her major problem. Her blood pressure during the first day on the floor was 85/46.

Nursing Diagnosis

The priorities and care plan changed from the time of the initial pre-clinical work to the days care was actually provided for this patient. Talking with nurses and doctors as well as talking with the patient (assessment) helped provide a better understanding of what her needs really were. Looking back, her chart was slightly confusing and even misleading. Initially, it appeared that a medical diagnosis of sepsis was a severe and grim, life-threatening problem for the patient. The initial care map for the patient going into the first day consisted of the following nursing diagnoses: 1) Infection related to unidentified microorganism as evidenced by a WBC count of 4.0, altered mental status, a temperature of 106 ° F, and lactic acid of 2.9; 2) Decreased Cardiac Output related to pathophysiology of medical illness as evidenced by a blood pressure of 85/46 on day one in the ICU and altered mental status; 3) Ineffective Tissue Perfusion related to impaired transport of oxygen, hypovolemia, interruption in blood flow, and decreased hemoglobin concentration in the blood as evidenced by oxygen saturation of 92% on room air, a hemoglobin of 9.5, a blood pressure of 85/46, and altered mental status; 4) Unstable Blood Glucose related to medical diagnosis of diabetes mellitus, BMI of 34.9, and disease process as evidenced by blood glucose readings of 154 and 184 and altered mental status; 5) Anxiety related to change in health status, environment, and self-concept as evidenced by restlessness, expressed concerns, and confusion (Gulanik & Myers, 2011).

After gaining information from the patient's chart before actually caring for her, Infection was deemed the priority nursing diagnosis because of her admitting medical diagnosis of sepsis. Also, when considering the pathophysiology of sepsis, especially within a hospital environment and for an older patient, its seriousness warranted attention. The initial goal going into the first day of caring for this patient was to help eradicate her infection by administering Zosyn, a broad spectrum antibiotic, while waiting for labs to identify the exact cause of the sepsis. Plans also included administering Levophed and isotonic normal saline to improve cardiac output and to improve tissue oxygenation by giving oxygen (Gulanik & Myers, 2011).

When stepping foot on the floor to care for this patient, the plan of care and the priorities changed. A more accurate picture of the patient's condition was obtained when her status was discussed with her doctor and nurses and with the patient herself. Infection was not the urgent problem. The patient was alert and oriented and was well hydrated according to the latest labs, and appeared ready for discharge. The only thing keeping her in the ICU was her unstable blood pressure. Practitioners were unable to wean her off the Levophed. Every time they tried to taper the dose down, her blood pressure dropped, as low as 65/48. It was perplexing why her blood pressure was so low. A specific microorganism was never identified as the cause of sepsis. The doctor explained that the infection could have been due to a complication as a result of her other chronic health conditions. The nurse added that the patient's other medications (particularly Thorazine and other antipsychotics) were likely causing her blood pressure to be so low.

After considering these updates in the patient's status and her improvement from the date of admission 3 days prior, her care plan was revised to address her current health problems. The infection appeared to be under control, as evidenced by an average temperature reading of 97 °F, a respiratory rate averaging 16/minute, a heart rate averaging in the 70s, and O2 sats averaging 100%. The patient was also alert and oriented. Deficient Fluid Volume and Decreased Cardiac Output became the priority nursing diagnoses. Deficient Fluid Volume related to infection, inadequate fluid intake, and failure of regulatory mechanisms as evidenced by hypotension and thirst was truly the major problem for this patient. The deficient fluid volume caused a decrease in cardiac output. Decreased Cardiac Output related to pathophysiology of medical illness as evidenced by a blood pressure of 85/46 on day one in the ICU and altered mental status was made the second most important problem. Pain, related to medical diagnosis of pancreatitis, as evidenced by verbal complaint of pain and grimacing upon palpation of the abdomen was the third most urgent problem. Ineffective Tissue Perfusion and Anxiety, as previously mentioned, were the fourth and fifth most urgent problems (Gulanik & Myers, 2011).

Ida Jean Orlando's Nursing Process Theory can be used to support the prioritization of the patient's needs as well as the interrelatedness of the aforementioned nursing diagnoses. Her theory states that the use of the nursing process by the nurse allows nursing care and actions to be deliberate rather than automatic. The theory defines professional nursing as "meeting the patient's needs for health care" (Johnson & Webber, 2010, p.135). The nursing process of assessment, diagnosis, planning, implementation, and evaluation allows the nurse to determine the patient's needs and to intervene appropriately to meet those needs (Johnson & Webber, 2010).

Applying the nursing process in caring for this patient is what caused the original care map to be revised. Deficient Fluid Volume, rather than Infection, was made the priority diagnosis. Assessment of the patient showed that the infection itself was well-controlled and that perhaps a separate disease process, such as a chronic condition was to blame for the poor fluid volume and subsequent low blood pressure. Recognizing the patient's low fluid volume and need for replacement allowed for appropriate nursing intervention. Correcting the volume deficit would fix the problem of Decreased Cardiac Output and any problems with poor tissue perfusion, which is why Deficient Fluid Volume was made the major diagnosis rather than Decreased Cardiac Output. Careful evaluation by the nurse (and nursing student) of the patient's response to nursing interventions and progress toward outcomes allowed for effective and purpose-driven nursing care. Assessing the patient continuously allowed for identification of her pain. By interacting with the patient through assessment and intervention, the nurse could meet the patient's need for pain relief. Further assessment by the nurse revealed patient anxiety and the fact that it was linked to her state of health. This allowed the nurse to understand that addressing the first four problems and interacting with the patient could help allay anxiety. As the nurse intervenes, revisions can be made to the plan of care in order to progress to meeting all health goals of the patient (Nursing Theory, 2011).

Outcomes

An expected outcome for this patient with Deficient Fluid Volume is that the patient will be normovolemic as evidenced by a SBP greater than or equal to 90 mmHg, a heart rate greater than or equal to 60 beats/min, and normal skin turgor within 24 hours of initiation of treatment. An expected outcome for this patient with Decreased Cardiac Output is that the patient will have adequate cardiac output within 24 hours of onset of treatment as evidenced by a SBP greater than or equal to 90 mmHg; a heart rate of greater than or equal to 60 beats/min; urine output of greater than 30 mL/hr; strong pulses in all extremities; warm, dry skin; clear lung sounds; and orientation to person, place, and time (Gulanik & Myers, 2011).

Interventions

There are numerous interventions that the nurse employs in caring for a patient with Deficient Fluid Volume. The most important interventions pertinent to this patient are encouraging her to drink fluids, administering parenteral fluids as ordered, and maintaining intravenous (IV) flow rates. Lack of fluid intake is a common cause of inadequate fluid volume (Gulanik & Myers, 2011). The patient did frequently state that she was thirsty, so oral hydration was provided in the form of water. Frequently offering drinks to the patient can help ensure that she gets the minimum 1600 mL/day of fluid (Campbell, 2011). The doctors had also ordered a continuous IV bolus infusion of 1000 mL 0.9% Normal Saline. Standard protocol for hypotension is 500-1000 mL boluses (American Medical Network, 2005). Normal saline is the crystalloid most often chosen for treatment of dehydration because it hydrates the vascular space. The fluid is isotonic to the body and therefore does not cause fluid to shift into or out of cells. It simply increases volume in the body (Winn, 2012).

Along with providing hydration for the patient, monitoring intake and output is an important nursing responsibility in managing the patient with deficient fluid volume. In the ICU at RMC, intake and output (I & O) is recorded on a flow sheet each hour of the shift. Both intake from medication drips, IV solutions, and oral fluids is recorded. This particular patient also had a Foley catheter, which allowed for easy assessment of output each hour. Both hourly and cumulative output was recorded. Typically, a urine output of less than 30 mL/hr is reported to the physician (Gulanik & Myers, 2011).

Research and Theory for Nursing Practice stated that there is no consensus regarding the best method for determining the necessary water intake of nursing home residents and older patients in general. Thirty mL/kg of body weight is one formula often used to ensure that patients are adequately hydrated, although the researchers said that it must be used with caution in patients who are extremely underweight or overweight. The researchers believed that of the four standards they examined, they recommend the one that encourages an intake of 75% of 1600 mL/m2 of body surface area because this standard provides the most individualized recommendation (Gaspar, 2011). Regardless of the formula used to ensure adequate fluid intake, it is imperative that the nurse monitor the dehydrated patient and the patient at risk for dehydration by ongoing assessment of I & O and other signs of dehydration (Collins, 2011).

Vasopressors were ordered for this patient to treat her low blood pressure as a result of deficient fluid volume. It is the nurse's responsibility to safely administer these potent drugs. This patient had an order for norepinephrine (Levophed), the most potent vasopressor. Levophed increases peripheral resistance by stimulating both alpha and beta1 adrenergic receptors. It is a positive inotrope and is often used to elevate the blood pressure when volume replacement is ineffective, such as in shock states or bacteremia. Levophed has fewer side effects than epinephrine, but it can occasionally produce anxiety, palpitations, and bradycardia (Hodgson & Kizior, 2011). Research has also shown that it has fewer side effects, such as cardiac dysrhythmias, than dopamine. In one study, it showed a 4% less mortality rate when used to treat shock compared to dopamine (De Backer, Biston, & Devriendt, 2010).

In conjunction with the hospital's sepsis protocol, Levophed was ordered at 4 mg/D5W 250 mL. Typically, it is ordered at 8 mg/500 mL D5W to run at 2-30 mcg/min for a mean arterial pressure (MAP) of greater than or equal to 65 (Regional Medical Center [RMC], 2012). The nurse thinks critically and calculates the drip rate for the patient. Levophed is administered in micrograms per minute. The original order came in milligrams/min. Four milligrams is equivalent to 4000 micrograms. Four thousand micrograms in 250 mL of D5W multiplied by 60 minutes equals 3.84 micrograms/minute. This is the rate for 1 mcg of Levophed. The nursing policy for the IV administration of Levophed states that 8 mg/500 mL is to be started at 2-10 mcg/min and to be increased by 1-2 mcg/min every 5-10 minutes (RMC, 2010). To administer 2 mcg/min, the nurse would take the available concentration of 4 mg/250 mL and compare it to the desired 2 mcg/min to be administered. Converting mcg into mg yields 0.002 mg. An equation would be set up where 4 mg/250 mL is equal to 0.002 mg/x, x being the desired rate in mL/hour. Cross multiplication gives 0.125 mL. Multiplying this by 60 minutes gives a rate of 7.5 mL/hr. The nurse would then set the pump for 7.5 mL/hr to give the patient 2 mcg/min of Levophed. The max dose is 30 mcg/min (RMC, 2010). The goal of treatment with

Levophed is to attain and maintain a SBP greater than or equal to 90 mmHg and a mean arterial pressure (MAP) greater than or equal to 65 (RMC, 2012).

The nurse must closely monitor the patient's blood pressure while administering this potent drug. RMC's policy is that the blood pressure be monitored non-invasively once at baseline and then every 15 minutes for one hour during initiation of treatment, followed by monitoring every 1 hour once the patient is stable (RMC, 2010). The dose of Levophed as well as the patient's blood pressure and MAP was documented hourly. Early in the morning (at 0700), she was on 3 mcg/min at a rate of 11.3 mL/hr. Her blood pressure was 125/66 with a MAP of 80. The next hour, she was bumped down to 2 mcg/min at a rate of 7.5 mL/hr. Her blood pressure decreased slightly to 115/59 with a MAP of 72. She was kept on 2 mcg/min for the next three hours. As her blood pressure and MAP remained unchanged, she was weaned to 1 mcg/min at a rate of 3.5 mL/hr, at which point her blood pressure dropped to 90/27 and her MAP to 40. At one point during the night when taken off the Levophed, her blood pressure dropped as low as 65/48. The doctor was notified. In the meantime, she was restarted on the drip at 2 mcg/min to bring her blood pressure back up.

When it was observed that the patient was not able to be successfully weaned off the Levophed, the doctor ordered Midodrine. Midodrine is also a vasopressor and is often used clinically as an orthostatic hypotensive adjunct. It works by forming an alpha1 agonist metabolite that stimulates alpha receptors in the vasculature, thus increasing blood pressure. For this patient, it was administered for its off-label uses—to treat hypotension related to infection and to treat hypotension induced by psychotropic agents (the patient was on several antipsychotic medications; Thorazine, in particular has been known to cause hypotension). The doctor thought that the antipsychotic meds, rather than the sepsis, were to blame for the patient's hypotension. Midodrine was ordered for 10 mg three times a day orally with meals. Nursing considerations for this drug were primarily to monitor blood pressure (Hodgson & Kizior, 2011).

Teaching was an important nursing intervention for this patient. Her deficient fluid volume and subsequent low blood pressure was the reason that she was being kept in the ICU. This was explained to her in laymen's terms. The potential complications of low blood pressure, such as poor tissue perfusion and organ dysfunction, as well as confusion and falling, were also explained. These explanations provided some anxiety relief to the patient, as she did not understand at first why she was being kept in the ICU. After patient teaching, she no longer appeared restless and no longer showed facial expressions of worry (grimacing, etc.). Also, the importance of staying hydrated at home was discussed with her. She was encouraged to drink plenty of water at home (Gulanik & Myers, 2011).

Many of the nursing interventions for the diagnosis of Decreased Cardiac Output are the same as for Deficient Fluid Volume. Correcting the lack of volume in the patient's system would subsequently correct the problem of decreased cardiac output in this case. Administration of isotonic saline, Levophed, and Midodrine, as well as calculating drip rates and monitoring blood pressure are all nursing responsibilities in treating poor cardiac output.

A few other, perhaps less complex interventions, are important as well. The administration of oxygen can be helpful to patients with Decreased Cardiac Output. This patient did have an order for oxygen via nasal cannula, which she was given one night when she became restless. Patient positioning can have an impact on cardiac output. The supine position at nighttime increased venous return for her, while encouraging her to be in a high-Fowler's or supine position during the daytime decreased preload and ventricular filling, thus improving oxygenation (Gulanik & Myers, 2011). Occasional lateral or side-lying positions are also effective at improving oxygenation. One study found that in obese patients with respiratory distress, prone positioning actually improved alveolar ventilation (Johnson & Meyenburg, 2009). Because this patient was able to reposition herself, she naturally assumed the most comfortable positions.

Promoting rest for this patient with Decreased Cardiac Output was another important nursing intervention employed while caring for her (Gulanik & Myers, 2011). She was confined to bed rest, but did receive assistance from physical therapy in moving from her bed to a chair and back to bed once a day. Drowsiness was a common side effect of many of the antipsychotic medications she received daily, such as Abilify (Hodgson & Kizior, 2011), which helped to promote rest and thus decrease her body's need for oxygen. Although this patient was able to bathe herself, assistance was provided to prevent overexertion (Gulanik & Myers, 2011).

Lastly, a cardiac diet was prescribed for the patient while she was in the hospital. Typically, cardiac diets are "healthier" than a regular diet and consist of no more than 25-35% fat, 50-60% carbohydrate, with limited cholesterol (no more than 200 mg/day) and sodium. It is also high in fiber, providing 20-30 g/day (Woodard, 2010).

Patient teaching concerning Decreased Cardiac Output consisted of explaining the physiologic process to the patient. She was taught that she needed medications to improve her blood pressure and fluids to improve the amount of volume in her body so that her heart could pump more effectively and thus better perfuse her organs (Gulanik & Myers, 2011).

Numerous aspects of culture were observed in caring for this patient. The African American culture in itself, as well as the broad culture of obesity was considered. Many African Americans are more prone to hypertension, in part because of a diet high in salt. There is also a high rate of obesity among African Americans because of poor diet and a sedentary lifestyle. The importance of making healthy choices about food was discussed with the patient. The cultural aspect of family was also explored, as nursing assessment included questioning about her home and family life. She was alone in the hospital and frequently expressed anxiety for her family members, which allowed the nurse and nursing student to act as a friend and advocate for her (Urden, Stacy, & Lough, 2010).

Evaluation

The patient's status improved greatly from the time of admission to the last day she was seen. She was alert and oriented, had an average temperature of 97.1, a WBC count of 5.2, a SBP well above 90 and a MAP well above 65 when on Levophed. The sepsis appeared to be under control, despite no identification of an exact cause. It would be safe to say that the goal of adequate fluid volume for this patient was partially met. Lab work, skin turgor, and urinary output showed that she was well hydrated and her heart rate was within normal limits. However, the ultimate goal of normovolemia was only partially met, as the patient was unable to maintain a safe blood pressure apart from the Levophed drip. Unfortunately, there was not enough clinical time to observe the long-term effect of Midodrine on her blood pressure.

Likewise, the desired outcome for the nursing diagnosis of Decreased Cardiac Output was partially met. According to the aforementioned criteria for this diagnosis, all were met except for the stipulation that SBP be greater than or equal to 90 mmHg.

The alternative plan for this patient was the Midodrine for blood pressure control. Perhaps her physicians will consider switching her to another drug other than Thorazine for treatment of her anxiety in order to alleviate problems with blood pressure. Once the patient's blood pressure is under control, she will be sent back to The Rehabilitation Center for further care. Although this patient may seem simple compared to other patients in the ICU, her ongoing care consists of managing her other chronic conditions.

Conclusion

This patient was admitted to RMC for altered mental status and fever. She was later diagnosed with acute sepsis, although lab work was inconclusive in determining a cause. The nursing student provided care for her on days 3 and 4 of her stay in the ICU, in which the main goal of nursing care was to wean her off Levophed while maintaining a safe blood pressure. Even with attention to her two main nursing diagnoses of Deficient Fluid Volume and Decreased Cardiac Output, the major goal of this patient's care was not fully met, perhaps due to other causes such as psychiatric meds and chronic conditions.

This client's case reveals that care of the critically ill patient requires astute attention and critical thinking on the nurse's part. A thorough knowledge of disease processes, regulation mechanisms within the human body, and pharmacology is imperative in managing patients such as this one. The importance of communication cannot be overlooked, as effective communication between the patient and members of the health care team were essential in promoting health for this patient. In all, the experience of caring for this patient was an eye-opening one as well as a good reminder to look at the big picture when caring for those who are critically ill.

References

American Medical Network. (2005). *Hypotension and shock treatment.* Retrieved from http://www.health.am/vein/more/hypotension_shock_treatment/Campbell N. (2011). Why is dehydration still a problem in healthcare? *Nursing Times, 107*(22), early online publication.

Regional Medical Center. (2010). *Administration of medications via intravenous infusion in adult patients, Policy #501.01A.*

Regional Medical Center. (2012). *Sepsis order set, 600-SOS-001.* Collins, M. (2011). Recognizing the face of dehydration. *Nursing,* August, 26-31.

De Backer, D., Biston, P., & Devriendt, J. (2010). Comparison of dopamine and norepinephrine in the treatment of shock. *New England Journal of Medicine, 362*(9), 779-789.

Gaspar, P.M. (2011). Comparison of four standards for determining adequate water intake of nursing home residents. *Research & Theory For Nursing Practice, 25*(1), 11-22. doi:10.1891/0889-7182.25.1.11

Gulanik, M. & Myers, J.L. (2011). *Nursing care plans: Diagnoses, interventions, and outcomes.* (7th ed.). St.Louis: Mosby-Elsevier.

Hodgson, B.B. & Kizior, R.J. (2011). Saunder's Nursing Drug

Handbook 2011. St.Louis, MO: Elsevier.

Johnson, B.M. & Webber, P.B. (2010). An introduction to theory and reasoning in nursing. (3rd ed.). Philadelphia, PA: Wolters Kluwer-Lippincott Williams & Wilkins.

Johnson, K.L. & Meyenburg, T. (2009). Physiological rationale and current evidence for therapeutic positioning of critically ill patients. *American Association of Critical Care Nurses, 20*(3), 228-240.

Nursing Theory. (2011). *Ida Jean Orlando's contribution to nursing theory: Deliberative nursing process.* Retrieved from http://nursing-theory.org/nursing-theorists/Ida-Jean-Orlando.php

Urden, L.D., Stacy, K.M., & Lough, M.E. (2010). *Critical care nursing: diagnosis and management.* St.Louis: Mosby-Elsevier.

Winn, L. (2012, October). *Endocrine.* Lecture at School of Nursing. City, State.

Woodard, L. (2010). Hospital Cardiac Diet. Retrieved from http://www.livestrong.com/article/224764-hospital-cardiac-diet/

Client Case Study

THE TRUTH ABOUT NURSING

Grading Criteria

Student: _____ Score: _____

Grading Criteria	Points	Faculty Comments	Points Awarded
Introduction Pt. Overview Scope of paper	 2 1		
Medical Diagnosis Dx for ICU adm. Patho Related S/S	 2 4 4		
Nursing Diagnosis 5 NANDA (1+ psych/soc) Priority with theorist support	 5 10		
Outcomes for top 2 NDX Appropriate for NDX Attainable within timeframe	#1 #2 2.5 2.5 2.5 2.5		
Interventions for top 2 NDX Interventions with rationale SOP /Clinical Path Patient/family teaching Critical Thinking Cultural Considerations	#1 #2 6 6 2 2 2 2 2 2 3		
Evaluation Progress toward outcomes Additional/alternative plan	#1 #2 5 5 1 1		

Conclusion Review of learning	3		
Grading Criteria	Points	Faculty Comments	Points Awarded

Sources
  5+ sources
  3+ primary nursing research
    Study results reviewed/applied
    Study poorly reviewed/applied
    Research omitted
	1
	3 3 3
	1 1 1
	0 0 0		

APA Format (Cover page, headings, margins, type size) **Format conforms to APA Format** **Format includes 1-3 APA errors** **Format includes 4-6 APA errors** **Format includes >6 errors**	 3 2 1 0		
APA- References/Reference Page **Conform to APA Format** **Include 1-3 APA errors** **Include 4-6 APA errors** **Include >6 APA errors** **Do not conform to APA**	4 3 2 1 0		

format			
Writing Style (Grammar, spelling, punctuation, language)			
Logical, organized, without errors	3		
Logical, organized minor errors (<5)	2		
Lacks logic/organization OR major spelling/grammar/errors (>5)	1		
Lacks logic / organization AND major spelling / grammar / errors (>5)	0		

Rebecca Parker

Transplant Paper: Kidney Transplantation

Fall 2012

Submitted in partial fulfillment of the requirements in the course

Adult Health Nursing III

Introduction

Overview

Organ transplantation is a medical procedure that offers hope to thousands of ill people. The procedure consists of surgically removing an organ (i.e., the heart, lung, pancreas, kidney, etc.) from one person and implanting it into another person. This gives the sick individual a new organ with the hope that it will adapt properly in its new body and perform its necessary functions in order to promote and restore health. There are many organizations that oversee the issues surrounding organ transplantation, including recipient and donor criteria, therapeutic regimens for post-transplant care, patient education, and research (Transplant Living, 2012).

Pathophysiology

Hypertension is a major cause of end-stage kidney disease (ESKD), which ultimately creates the need for a kidney transplant.

Hypertension, or high blood pressure, is defined as a systolic blood pressure (BP) greater than or equal to 140 mmHg and/or a diastolic BP greater than or equal to 90 mmHg. It has numerous risk factors and causes, including older age (greater than 65 years old), stress, a high-salt diet, and obesity. Kidney problems such as tumors and problems of the renal cortex and medulla can also contribute to the development of hypertension (Ignatavicius & Workman, 2011).

A system of checks and balances works within the body to maintain a normal BP (120/80 or less). One of these mechanisms is arterial baroreceptors. These receptors are found in the heart and are able to sense changes in arterial blood pressure. They control changes in BP through actions of the vagus nerve. For some unknown reason, these baroreceptors fail in hypertension. The body also controls BP by sensing shifts in fluid volume. If there is too much water and/or sodium in the body, which increases cardiac output, the kidneys are able to detect this and increase urinary output (diuresis). The renin-angiotensin-aldosterone system (RAAS) also keeps BP in check. The enzyme renin, produced by the kidneys, starts a process in the body that controls aldosterone release and hence BP. For some reason, in hypertension, renin is improperly secreted. Lastly, vascular autoregulation is impaired in hypertension. Prolonged periods of high blood pressure cause thickening of arteriole walls, which can lead to kidney failure and cardiac problems (Ignatavicius & Workman, 2011).

Recipient Criteria

Physical criteria

An individual in need of a kidney transplant must meet strict criteria in order to be considered. ESKD is typically the reason a patient would need a new kidney. ESKD is defined as a glomerular filtration rate (GFR) of less than 15 mL/min (normal is 100 mL/min). Because of poor GFR, waste products such as urea and creatinine build up in the blood. Kidney function is so poor that the patient cannot survive without treatment. ESKD is preceded by chronic kidney disease (CKD), a progressive deterioration of kidney function. In the early stages of CKD, GFR is normal; in severe CKD GFR is between 15 and 29 mL/min. In ESKD, because of the buildup of waste products in the blood, electrolyte and acid-base imbalances occur (Ignatavicius & Workman, 2011).

The patient with end-stage kidney disease has a remarkable clinical presentation. The individual has typically been on dialysis for some time because kidney function is so poor. Nearly every system of the body is affected by the non-functioning kidneys. Urine output is significantly reduced if not absent and thus urine osmolarity is fixed. The patient experiences fluid overload, evidenced by edema, hypertension, and electrolyte disturbances. The patient is hyperkalemic because the body is unable to excrete potassium. Serum potassium levels can rise to 7 mEq/L. Paresthesias, muscle weakness, and disturbances in the heart's electrical conduction system can occur. The patient is also metabolically acidotic because of the inability to excrete hydrogen ions. He often presents with Kussmaul respirations in an attempt to excrete excess carbon dioxide. Respiratory alkalosis follows. The body also retains phosphorus, which subsequently causes a drop in serum calcium levels. Parathyroid hormone stimulates the bones to release more calcium into the blood, which causes poor bone density and an increased risk of fractures. Crystals form in the body once the calcium-phosphorus level reaches 70 mg/dL and they can deposit in the joints, lungs, and other organs. They can also form on the skin, causing extreme pruritis and discomfort (Ignatavicius & Workman, 2011).

The patient in ESKD also experiences anemia (hemoglobin less than 12 gm/dL), as the kidneys are unable to produce erythropoietin necessary for red blood cell production. Heart failure can result from hypertension and fluid overload. Bad breath is another sign of ESKD, as the normal flora of the mouth is altered due to waste product build-up in the blood (Ignatavicius & Workman, 2011).

Specific criteria exist for individuals in need of a kidney transplant. Typically, patients are between 2 and 70 years old (although those outside these ranges can receive transplants too). The person must be free of illnesses that could directly complicate a transplanted kidney, such as advanced heart disease and chronic respiratory infections and diseases, as a new kidney could make these conditions worse. Patients with ESKD who also have late stages of cancer are recommended for dialysis rather than renal transplant, but may apply for a new kidney once they have been cancer-free for 2 years. Those with chronic infections are also excluded, as immunosuppressant medications needed for successful transplantation may worsen these conditions (Ignatavicius & Workman, 2011). Those with viral infections, such as HIV, hepatitis, and cytomegalovirus are not likely to be chosen for a kidney transplant, as the presence of these viruses predisposes them to poor recovery (National Kidney Federation [NKF], 2011). Individuals who also have diabetes mellitus and other endocrine issues are eligible for transplants, but must be closely monitored. Urinary tract problems as well as gastrointestinal problems must be corrected and treated before the patient is deemed an eligible organ recipient (Ignatavicius & Workman, 2011).

Psychosocial criteria

Lastly, individuals who abuse alcohol or drugs are excluded from receiving a new kidney (Ignatavicius & Workman, 2011).

Donor Criteria

Physical criteria

There are different types of organ donors, including living related and unrelated donors, non-heart-beating donors, and cadaver donors. Qualified individuals who wish to donate an organ are usually between the ages of 18 and 70 years old. They are generally healthy, with no chronic illnesses such as diabetes mellitus, heart disease, HIV, sickle cell disease, hypertension, or kidney disease. An individual who wants to donate a kidney can call the Living Kidney Donor Program to obtain a questionnaire. If this initial screening clears, the process can continue. The potential donor is contacted by a nurse coordinator. The individual goes to a hospital where transplants take place in order to have blood drawn. Blood type, antigen type, and cross match are evaluated to determine whether the kidney will work for a potential recipient. The potential donor is then extensively examined. A general health assessment is performed, which includes urine testing, blood testing, CT scanning, angiograms, and EKGs. These tests help determine kidney function, anatomy, and overall health (University of Maryland Medical Center [UMMC], 2012).

Individuals who wish to donate an organ once they die can ensure this happens by registering in their state of residence to become an organ donor (National Kidney Registry, 2012). Once the person has died, their kidney is immediately removed (Ignatavicius & Workman, 2011). Many of the same criteria exist for deceased donors as for living donors when it comes to donating a kidney. The deceased individual, often a victim of a motor vehicle accident or a substantial fall, is typically overall healthy before the traumatic incidence that caused death. Deceased donors are normally young, between the ages of 10 and 39 years old, have normal kidney function and no chronic or transmissible diseases at the time of death. The recipient 3-year survival rate is slightly lower for kidneys coming from a deceased donor (94%) compared to those coming from a living donor (97-98%) (The Rogosin Institute, 2012).

Psychosocial criteria

Some transplant centers perform psychiatric assessments on potential donors to determine their reason for donating (Ignatavicius & Workman, 2011). Many transplant organizations and centers discuss psychosocial implications with donors to make them aware of physical, financial, and psychological implications of kidney donation (UMMC, 2012).

Therapeutic Management

Organ rejection

Ten to twenty percent of kidney transplant recipients experience rejection of the new organ. Most rejection episodes occur within the first 6 months after the transplant (Columbia University Medical Center, 2012). Kidney rejections are classified as either hyperacute, acute or chronic (Ignatavicius & Workman,

2011).

A hyperacute kidney rejection occurs within 48 hours of the transplant and is evidenced by increased temperature and blood pressure as well as pain at the site. Treatment is immediate removal of the kidney (Ignatavicius & Workman, 2011).

Acute kidney rejection has a sudden onset and is both more common and easier to treat than chronic rejection. It is caused by the body's white blood cells attacking the new kidney or from an attack of newly formed antibodies against the kidney. Signs and symptoms of acute kidney rejection are creatinine levels that do not decrease after the transplant or that decrease and then rise again; fever of over 100 degrees Fahrenheit; chills, vomiting, and other flu-like symptoms; weight gain of 2-4 pounds a week; systemic edema; and decreased urinary output (Cleveland Clinic, 2012). Ultrasounds and Doppler scans help to determine if there is reduced blood flow to the new kidney (NKF, 2012). Repeated complete blood counts (CBC) also help to determine if rejection is taking place (Cleveland Clinic, 2012). Kidney biopsy is considered the best diagnostic tool for determining the presence of acute rejection. Acute kidney rejection is treated with intravenous (IV) methylprednisolone, a high-dose immunosuppressant, over the course of three days. If this drug is not effective at treating the rejection, the patient will be given other anti-rejection drugs, such as tacrolimus and microphenalate, which are stronger than the ones initially prescribed. Anti-thrombocyte globulin and OKT3 antibody are the last drugs of choice to treat acute rejection, since they can have severe side effects such as pulmonary edema and shortness of breath, although they do have a 70% success rate (NKF, 2012).

Chronic kidney rejection occurs months to years after the transplant and is marked by a gradual decline in kidney function. The creatinine level and BUN start to rise in the blood, which ultimately causes fluid and electrolyte disturbances (Ignatavicius & Workman, 2011). The patient's initial anti-rejection meds can be traded for stronger meds such as tacrolimus and microphenalate, but these are toxic to the kidneys in this type of rejection (NKF, 2012). Management of this patient is supportive until dialysis is needed and a second kidney transplanted is warranted (Ignatavicius & Workman, 2011).

The main nursing responsibility concerning kidney rejection is monitoring the patient for any signs and symptoms of rejection. Strict measurement of intake and output is essential in kidney transplant patients, and is made simpler by the use of a Foley catheter. Urine output should be assessed closely for the first 48 hours postoperatively for amount and color. A sudden decrease in urinary output could signal problems with the new kidney. Urine should be pink to red for the first few days or weeks and then return to its normal yellow-straw color. Urine specimens may also be ordered for tracking of glucose measurement and urinalysis. Daily weights and blood pressure checks every 2 to 4 hours postoperatively are important to assess fluid status and circulation. Serum electrolytes, particularly sodium and potassium, should be monitored to assess functioning of the new kidney (Ignatavicius & Workman, 2011).

Immunosuppression

A number of medications are used to promote optimal outcomes for patients who receive a kidney transplant. Immunosuppressants are drugs that are used to prevent the patient's body from having an adverse reaction to the new kidney that could lead to organ rejection (Ignatavicius & Workman,

2011).

Methylprednisolone is classified as a steroid and is used primarily to decrease inflammation in patients with kidney transplants. It works by suppressing the migration of white blood cells to the operative site and reverses capillary permeability. It is available in oral, intramuscular (IM) and IV preparations. Steroid medications have many unpleasant side effects. Methylprednisolone may cause anxiety, insomnia, and mood swings. It also increases the risk of infection because it suppresses the immune system. It may also cause weight gain, facial flushing, and acne. It is important for nurses to perform a baseline assessment to obtain blood pressure, weight, serum glucose, and electrolytes. During treatment with this medication, the nurse should monitor the patient's intake and output, bowel pattern, serum electrolytes (especially calcium and potassium), and for any signs of infection. It is imperative that the nurse inform the patient to not abruptly stop taking this medication because of the risk of adrenal insufficiency (Hodgson & Kizior, 2011).

Tacrolimus is another medication frequently used to prevent rejection of a new kidney. It is also an immunosuppressant and works by binding to proteins within cells to halt T-lymphocyte activation. Phosphotase activity is blocked and the immune system complex is unable to progress in causing organ rejection. Tacrolimus is indicated as prophylaxis for organ rejection and is often given in conjunction with adrenal corticosteroids and azathioprine or mycophenolate. It is metabolized in the liver and excreted in stool and cannot be removed by dialysis. It can be given orally or by injection. Side effects include headache, tremor, tingling sensation in the limbs, constipation/diarrhea, and hypertension. Neprhotoxicity, neurotoxicity, and pleural effusion can occur. Nurses should assess the patient's renal function and use of any other immunosuppressants. An aqueous solution of epinephrine as well as oxygen should be at the bedside before IV infusion is begun. Labs, including serum creatinine, potassium, and CBC with differential should be monitored. The patient should be advised to avoid sun exposure while on this medication to reduce the risk of a photosensitivity reaction (Hodgson & Kizior, 2011).

Azathioprine is another immunosuppressant used to prevent kidney rejection. This medication works by inhibiting DNA, RNA, and protein synthesis. It suppresses the immune cells responsible for hypersensitivity reactions. It is available as oral and intravenous preparations. Side effects include nausea, vomiting, and poor appetite as well as an occasional rash. Use of this medication, as with all immunosuppressants, predisposes the individual to infection, so the nurse should assess white blood cell counts and implement measures to prevent infection, such as assisting the patient with thorough hygiene and handwashing. Results of hepatic function studies should also be examined since hepatotoxicity is a possible adverse reaction (Hodgson & Kizior, 2011).

Nursing research

A recent study published by the *British Journal of Nursing* found that nurses do not have sufficient knowledge about immunosuppressive agents used for kidney transplants. Data was collected from 50 nurses working with kidney transplant patients on three different wards in a Singapore hospital. A 30 question questionnaire was given to test nurses' knowledge of immunosuppressive drugs used for kidney transplant patients. Questions were true or false and were related to indications, identification, interactions, drug administration, drug monitoring, and adverse effects. A score of 70% was considered to show that the nurse had adequate knowledge of immunosuppressive agents. Results showed that only 46% of the nurses received the 70% score. The data also showed that nurses who attended the yearly lecture on kidney transplant medications actually obtained lower scores than nurses who did not attend. More experience and postgraduate education were not associated with higher scores.

The implications of this study are that nurses need more education concerning these immunosuppressant medications for kidney transplant patients in order to safely practice nursing. The authors recommend that nurse education programs become accredited for these nurses and that more effective teaching strategies be used; that nurses attend these programs every 6 months instead of once a year; and that more emphasis be placed on lifelong career learning (Mohamad, Yang, Jin, Lee, & Yin, 2012).

Nutrition

The diet of patients with kidney transplants should be individualized for optimal outcomes. Generally, in the period before transplantation, the patient may have low visceral protein stores and have deficits of vitamin B6, folic acid, iron, vitamin C and vitamin D. The goal of nutrition therapy prior to transplant surgery is to correct these deficits. Immediately following transplantation, energy needs are very high and the patient should consume 30-35 kcal/kg. About 6 weeks after the surgery, energy needs may return to the patient's baseline energy requirements. Protein needs are also high initially after surgery and protein should therefore not be restricted. Glucose intolerance may develop as a result of medications and weight gain is common after transplantation, which further necessitates an overall healthy diet (Grodner, Long, & Walkingshaw, 2007).

A heart-healthy diet low in fat and cholesterol is recommended over the long run. Patients should also be conscious of their sodium intake. A diet rich in fruits, vegetables, and complex carbohydrates is recommended. Because potassium, calcium, and phosphorus levels may vary with the medications, specific instruction should be individualized for each patient (National Kidney Foundation, 2010).

Discharge Teaching

Weight gain is a major problem for post kidney transplant

patients. Results of a study by *Progress in Transplantation* showed that steroids given to patients after transplantation cause them to crave sweets and have a larger appetite, that patients feared too much physical activity could "mess up" their new kidney, and that these patients felt embarrassment and frustration about their weight gain. Participants in this study believed that written instructions on meal plans would be helpful in eating a healthy diet, that a support group of other people who had received kidney transplants would provide moral support, and that continued support from doctors and nurses would be beneficial if continued for years after the transplant (Stanfill, Bloodworth, & Cashion, 2012).

Nursing research

The *Nephrology Nursing Journal* published a phenomenological study in 2011 that explored the feelings and education needs of patients in the post-surgery phase of kidney transplantation. Semi-structured interviews were performed on 10 post-transplant patients ranging in ages from 41 to 66 years. The interviews were done between days 7 and 21 of the transplant operation. Patients reported numerous feelings, which were summed up as feeling "torn." The first few weeks after transplantation, patients reflected on the comparison between dialysis and a new kidney and were hopeful that the transplant would bring the desired changes to promote quality of life. Over the next few weeks, if the transplant had been successful, patients reported feelings of joy and gratitude to the donor. Patients described their pain associated with the new kidney right after surgery and the feelings of uncertainty about the new kidney being able to perform its role and how this placed more responsibility on them to care for themselves properly. Many patients reported optimism over their new found independence. A major concern for post-transplant patients was the need for support systems and advice regarding self-care, diet, medications, rehabilitation programs, and return to work (Wiederhold, Langer, & Landenberger, 2011).

The authors considered the patients' expressed concerns and created practical solutions to patient education needs. To help patients cope with psycho-emotional problems, nurses can assist patients with empowerment, emotional support, and reality orientation (Wiederhold, Langer, & Landenberger, 2011). Patients who feel that they have a strong support system experience a greater quality of life after kidney transplantation than those who do not have support (White & Gallagher, 2010). To address knowledge deficits, nurses should teach post-transplant patients how to monitor their intake and output and develop a personalized diet plan. For medically related knowledge deficits, nurses should teach patients how to identify complications with the transplant and how to respond to them; physical limitations following the transplant; medication indications, interactions, and side effects (including written materials); and practical advice for promoting a healthy lifestyle. Nurses should also instruct these patients about exercise options and continence training. Lastly, nurses should provide information concerning financial support and job rehabilitation after the transplant (Wiederhold, Langer, & Landenberger, 2011).

A study by the *International Journal of Nursing Practice* further demonstrates the importance of patient education in regard to kidney transplantation. This pilot study of 100 kidney transplant patients of at least 6 months post-op assessed their compliance in several areas of instruction. Ninety-seven percent of patients were compliant with their immunosuppressant medication regimen.

Reasons given for non-compliance to other medications included forgetfulness, feeling better without taking the medication, deeming the medication unimportant, and unpleasant side effects. While roughly 67% of patients did follow a low fat diet, just 31% adhered to a low-salt diet. Reasons given for non-adherence to the prescribed diet included dislike of the diet, lack of knowledge of the diet, and financial difficulties. Most patients did attend their nephrology follow-up appointments and scheduling conflicts with work was the main reason given for missing appointments. Other areas to include in patient teaching according to this article include advising the patient to avoid overcrowded areas, to bathe daily, to avoid sun exposure, to walk for exercise, to perform self-breast exams (in women), and to quit smoking. Overall, the study showed that there is a high rate of non-compliance in kidney transplant patients. The implications of this study are that nurses need to continually assess the learning needs of their patient populations; provide effective and meaningful teaching strategies; and offer continual follow-up assessment, instruction, and encouragement to improve compliance (Gheith, El-Saadany, Abuo Donia, & Salem, 2008).

Conclusion

Kidney transplantation is a wonderful treatment for failing kidneys. However, in order for a patient to reap all its benefits, both he or she and the nurse must work together. The nurse must be aware of pathophysiological problems that lead to kidney transplantation and help the patient prevent worsening kidney function (Ignatavicius & Workman, 2011). Nurses must be knowledgeable about medications used to treat patients with kidney transplants in order to provide safe care and effective patient education (Mohamad, Yang, Jin, Lee, & Yin, 2012). Patient teaching is perhaps one of the most important roles of the nurse, as knowledge allows the patient to take control of his health and improves patient outcomes. The registered nurse is also an invaluable source of support and acts as an advocate for the patient in all aspects of life both pre, intra, and post renal transplantation (Wiederhold, Langer, & Landenberger, 2011).

References

Cleveland Clinic. (2012). *Transplant programs.* Retrieved from http://my.clevelandclinic.org/transplant/services/kidney/what_you_need_to_know.aspx

Columbia University Medical Center. (2012). *Renal and pancreatic transplant.* Retrieved from http://www.columbiasurgery.org/pat/kidneypancreastx/rejection.html

Gheith, O., El-Saadany, S., & Abuo Donia, S., & Salem, Y. (2008). Compliance of kidney transplant patients to the recommended lifestyle behaviours: single centre experience. *International Journal of Nursing Practice, 14*(5), 398-407.

Grodner, M., Long, S., & Walkingshaw, B.C. (2007). *Foundations and Clinical Applications of Nutrition.* St.Louis, MO: Mosby-Elsevier.

Hodgson, B.B. & Kizior, R.J. (2011). Saunder's Nursing Drug Handbook 2011. St.Louis, MO: Elsevier.

Ignatavicius, D.D. & Workman, M.L. (2011*). Medical-surgical nursing: patient-centered collaborative care.* (6th ed). St.Louis, MO: Mosby.

Mohamad, M., Yang, L., Jin, X., Lee, P.T., & Yin, T.K. (2012). Knowledge of immunosuppressive drugs used in kidney transplants. *British Journal of Nursing, 21*(13), 795-800.

National Kidney Federation. (2011). *Can everyone on dialysis have a kidney transplant.* Retrieved from http://www.kidney.org.uk/Medical-Info/transplant/txhave.html

National Kidney Federation (2012). *What is transplant rejection.* Retrieved from http://www.kidney.org.uk/Medical-Info/transplant/txrej.html

National Kidney Foundation. (2010). *Nutrition and Transplantation.* Retrieved from *www.kidney.org/atoz/pdf/nutri_trans.pdf*

National Kidney Registry. (2012). *I'm considering donating my kidney. I want to donate when I pass away.* Retrieved from http://www.kidneyregistry.org/pass_donate.php

Stanfill, A., Bloodworth, R., & Cashion, A. (2012). Lessons learned: experiences of gaining weight by kidney transplant recipients. *Progress in Transplantation, 22*(1), 71-78. doi:10.7182/pit2012986

The Rogosin Institute. (2012). *Deceased/living donor kidney transplantation.* Retrieved from http://rogosin.org/treatment-areas/treatment-transplantation/treatment-deceased-donor-kidney-transplant.php

Transplant Living. (2012). *Frequently asked questions.* Retrieved from http://www.transplantliving.org/community/patient-resources/frequently-asked-questions/

University of Maryland Medical Center. (2012). *Transplant Center.* Retrieved from http://www.umm.edu/transplant/lkd_eval_process.htm

White, C. & Gallagher, P. (2010). Effect of patient coping preferences on quality of life following renal transplantation. *Journal of Advanced Nursing, 66*(11), 2550-2559. doi: 10.1111/j.1365-2648.2010. 05410. x

Wiederhold, D., Langer, G., & Landenberger, M. (2011). Ambivalent lived experiences and instruction needs of patients in the early period after kidney transplantation: A phenomenological study. *Nephrology Nursing Journal, 38*(4), 417-423.

Transplant Paper Evaluation Form

Criteria / Points	Comments	Points
Introduction 　Overview (5) 　Patho (5)		
Recipient Criteria 　Physical criteria (5) 　Psychosocial criteria (5)		
Donor Criteria 　Physical criteria (5) 　Psychosocial criteria (5)		
Therapeutic Management 　Organ rejection (15) 　Immunosuppression (10) 　Nutrition (5)		
Discharge teaching (10)		
Nursing Research (15) Study reviewed & applied Study poorly reviewed or applied Study poorly reviewed and poorly applied Research omitted	3 studies required 5　5　5 3　3　3 1　1　1 0　0　0	
Conclusion (5)		
APA Format (Cover page,		

headings, margins, type) Format conforms to APA Includes 1-3 APA errors Has 4-6 APA errors Format has >6 errors	3 2 1 0	
APA- References/Reference Page Conforms to APA Format Includes 1-3 APA errors Includes 4-6 APA errors Includes >6 APA errors Do not conform to APA format	4 3 2 1 0	
Writing Style (Grammar, spelling, punctuation, language) Logical, organized, without errors Logical, organized minor errors (<5) Lacks logic/organization **OR** major spelling / grammar/errors (>5) Lacks logic / organization **AND** major spelling / grammar / errors (>5)	3 2 1 0	
Comments:	Grade:	

Rebecca Parker

Disability Study

Spring 2013

Submitted in partial fulfillment of the requirements in the course

Nursing Care of the Rehabilitation Client

Introduction

For this assignment, I chose to act as a paraplegic. This

particular disability was chosen after reading and thinking about potential difficulties faced by one with hemiplegia, paraplegia, and quadriplegia. I determined that being a paraplegic would require the least assistance. I chose to have no use of my legs, figuring that for the day's activities I would be just fine as long as I had use of my arms. This would still allow for activities such as typing, wheeling myself, and eating, etc.

Experience with the Disability

This assignment went pretty much as I expected. With just several hours in the wheelchair, I did; however, gain some insight into the life of a paraplegic and the unique challenges one with this disability faces. When we picked the wheelchair up from school, my peers and I noticed immediately how heavy and bulky it was. It was difficult to fit it into the SUV and we even had to put two of the seats down and maneuver it a special way to get it to fit into the car. This made me think that a bigger car is needed for those in a wheelchair.

It was difficult to fulfill my role as a paraplegic. In the car, I noticed that I had been moving my feet in order to cross them at the ankles and rotating my ankles just to keep things lose. When realizing this, I had to remind myself that a paraplegic would not be able to move the legs voluntarily and with the ease that I did. I suddenly became aware of how often I move my feet and legs, even just when sitting.

The first place we went was to Target. I immediately felt like a burden to Amelia and Britt, as I was the slow-moving one and the last out of the car. They had to retrieve the awkwardly placed, heavy wheelchair from the trunk and bring it around to the side of the car. It was not too difficult to get into the chair by myself, as I was able to use the handle inside the car for stability and gravity to help with moving down into the chair. I wheeled myself from the car to the inside of the store. By the time I got inside the store, my arms were tired from wheeling, and I had Britt wheel me from there. An interesting observation was that while sitting in the wheelchair, I was not able to reach items that were much above waist-level on the shelves. I would have needed a reacher or some other adaptive device in order to do this.

It was not too difficult to be wheeled through the aisles, as the store was not crowded and the aisles were big enough for the wheelchair to fit. As Britt wheeled me down a shoe aisle, a woman with her cart saw us coming and quickly moved it out of the aisle. I am guessing this was out of politeness. During our time in Target, I neither felt over noticed nor overlooked. I think overall, people that saw me in the wheelchair saw me as just a normal person.

We went to the Starbucks inside Target before leaving. The cashier was just as friendly to me in the wheelchair as I think she would have been if I had not been in the wheelchair. It was easy to swipe my gift card at the counter. When my drink was ready, Britt had to hold it so that I could wheel myself over to the other table in order to put cream in it. I imagine it would have been difficult to wheel myself while trying to hold coffee in one hand.

By the time we left Target, it was raining outside. Getting into the car was much more difficult than getting out of it, as I had to pull myself up to get in. I grabbed the overhead handle in the car as well as the handle on the door of the car to pull up. I had to constantly remind myself that I was not allowed to use my legs. I imagine that some paraplegics must have a lot of upper body strength to compensate for no use of the legs. Again, I felt like a nuisance as my friends had to stand in the rain while I transferred and then once again haul the bulky wheelchair back into the trunk.

Next, we went to downtown to the mall. Amelia, the driver, had to think strategically about the best place to park in the parking garage. Ideally, she looked for a spot that was not too far from the entrance as well as one that was not next to other vehicles, as this would have made it harder to squeeze the wheelchair between two cars. She did pretty well with this. I managed to get out of the car the same way as before. Amelia wheeled me to the ramp just outside the entrance to the food court. It was a little scary for me to be wheeled down the ramp, as speed picked up. I came to appreciate the presence of the ramp, as it would have been nearly impossible to use the few available stairs to get down into the food court.

I did feel like an odd ball, as this area of the mall was busy at the time we entered. I needed to use the restroom, so Amelia pushed me into the family bathroom that had a handicap sign on the wall just outside it. If she had not been with me, it would have been very difficult to get into the bathroom stall, as it was a normal door with no "easy" button to open it. I can certainly see how toileting would be a tremendous challenge for a person with this type of disability. I did cheat by using my legs and feet to get onto the toilet, but realizing that this would not be possible for a person with real paralysis. This again brought attention to the idea of feeling like a burden, as toileting would certainly require more help. Amelia stood by to open the door for me.

We went to Barnes and Noble in order to sit and do schoolwork. A few people looked up as we wheeled by, but I did not notice any rude stares. My peers made special accommodations for me to sit at the end of a table by rearranging several chairs. It seemed like way too much work to try to sit me anywhere else because space was tight. Before we left the mall, I revisited the same restroom, but this time without assistance from my partners. Two moms with their young children were in the bathroom and actually held the door for me to get into the stall. They were also quick to move their strollers out of the way to make space for me. I found them to be very kind, polite, and helpful.

To address the challenges I faced in the wheelchair, I think more doors, especially bathroom doors/stalls should have buttons for handicap people to press in order to get in and out more easily. Also, I think having a lighter weight wheelchair would help to at least lighten the job of the caregiver. I think it would be difficult to make all items in a store easily accessible for someone in a wheelchair, but perhaps stores could provide reachers for these individuals when they first enter the store to at least make the shopping experience a little easier.

Perceptions of Incontinence Product

For this experience, the incontinence product worn was a small/medium-sized Depend Silhoutte for Women. I only noticed that it seemed to bunch a few times, which was nothing more than slightly annoying. It was not obvious by looking at my jeans that I was wearing this brief. I really did not notice it was there most of the time. I can imagine; however, that on a hot day it might be uncomfortable to wear such a product, as it might cause one to sweat more.

The Depend did become significantly more annoying and uncomfortable once it was wet (with roughly 30 mL of water). It became cold and made me feel like I did not want to move. This experience reaffirmed for me what I believed previously believed about incontinence. After sitting in a wet brief for just 30 minutes, I understand the importance of prompt perineal hygiene for those who are incontinent, as the dampness is irritating to the skin and is a perfect environment for the growth of unpleasant microorganisms.

I think it would be a terrible thing to be incontinent. My brief was only soiled with a small amount of water; for those with true incontinence, their briefs are soiled more frequently, with more liquid, and with actual urine. This has greater implications for skin integrity, clothing choices, and social acceptance (I know this from my experience of working in a nursing home). Also, for those with paraplegia or other physical limitations, extensive assistance is needed for proper perineal hygiene.

Experience as a Helper

The experience as a helper was very similar to what I had expected. Trying to wheel my partner through the checkout line at Starbucks was slightly challenging, as space was limited. I again noticed that transporting the wheelchair into and out of the car was harder than I originally expected. It is heavy and bulky! During the experience, I did see myself as a helper and as someone there to assist my "disabled" friend. I did notice several looks from strangers. Some looked perplexed; I wondered if they knew we were actors. I found it surprising that while exiting Starbucks, the man sitting by the door did not offer to open it for us even though he could see that I was having a hard time holding the door and pushing the wheelchair. On a more positive note, a driver that was trying to park next to our car decided not to because he saw that Brittany was in a wheelchair and needed more space to get in. I interpreted this as courtesy. Brittany's attitude was the same as it had been when she was the helper. She did not seem frustrated, and even once mentioned that she thought the wheelchair was comfortable.

From this experience, I can truly understand how family members of physically disabled individuals burn out. It is both physically and emotionally tiring to care for someone in a wheelchair. Simple activities are much more difficult to perform and everything seems to take longer when in a wheelchair or caring for one in a wheelchair. Being a caregiver is certainly a challenging role!

Conclusion

Being in a wheelchair for whatever reason presents numerous challenges, such as transferring, accessibility, and self-care. Incontinence products are helpful in managing incontinence, but should be changed promptly when soiled, as they quickly become uncomfortable. Acting as an aide to one in a wheelchair is also difficult and requires patience and understanding.

Case Study: Fanconi Anemia & Preimplantation Testing

(Names of Group Members)

Submitted in partial fulfillment of the requirements in the course

Transition to Professional Nursing Practicum

Genetic selection is a heavily debated topic and in cases like Molly Nash's, many ethical issues are raised. Molly was a six-year-old girl with Fanconi anemia in need of a stem cell transplant. For this reason, her parents conceived a child who was genetically selected to be a perfect match for Molly so that she could receive a life-saving bone marrow transplant. This case was very unique because it was the first time anyone genetically selected their children, for the benefit of someone else. The purpose of this paper is to critically examine the ethical issues surrounding the case of Molly Nash. There are advantages and disadvantages to genetic selection and nurses take on responsibility when caring for families who are debating this process. It is a difficult decision to make but parents will go to great lengths to save their children (Frankenfieled, 2000).

Pro Perspective

There are many benefits of preimplantation genetic testing (PGD) and in vitro fertilization (IVF). Molly Nash benefited greatly from the birth of her brother and the genetic selection that went along with it. Molly's brother, Adam, was not harmed in any way when donating stem cells from his umbilical blood to his sister. He is helping her live a happier life dealing with her Fanconi anemia. He is also increasing her survival rate to 85% just because he is her sibling. The selected traits were not only good for Molly, but also good for Adam. The Nash family will not have to worry about their son Adam having Fanconi anemia and they will be a little more at ease knowing that their daughter, Molly, will have a better chance at a happier and healthier life (Frankenfield, 2000).

Genetic selection such as in this case can be tricky, but if it can make a family happier and help someone who is in dire need of a transplant to increase their chance of survival, then perhaps it is justified. Also, picking an embryo that does not have a debilitating disease that runs in one's family is good for that unborn child and also for the parents of that child. The parents will not have to worry about their child going through a hard time and suffering from whatever genetic disease he or she may be at risk for (Frankenfield, 2000).

Con Perspective

In addition to the many benefits of preimplantation testing, there are several disadvantages as well. First and foremost, selecting traits for a child diminishes the natural joy and surprise of conception and childbirth. By choosing desirable characteristics for a baby, that baby will be born for the benefit of another and therefore certain outcomes are expected of that child. For example, in the case of the Nash family, Adam was born with the job of saving his sister's life after his genetic traits were hand-picked. Furthermore, when a child is born with a specific purpose, that child has the potential to become abandoned or neglected once his or her job is fulfilled, such as after the retrieval of stem cells (Frankenfield, 2000).

Another drawback of preimplantation trait selection is the trial and error component. By making the conscious choice to select the genetic characteristics of an embryo, it becomes necessary to destroy other unwanted embryos which do not meet the requirements set forth by the family. If life does indeed begin at conception, this raises the ethical dilemma of murder in regard to those unwanted embryos and whether or not any stage of life should be disposable (Simoncelli, 2003).

Nursing Responsibilities

Nurses play a huge role in helping couples with a serious genetic disorder consider who are considering PGD. Since nurses are one of the front-line resources, they should provide adequate information about the benefits and limitations of this type of testing as well as educate and assist couples who consider PGD and IVF. According to the National Institution of Health, nurses and other health care providers can also assist couples by anticipating ethical concerns and supporting research surrounding the use of PGD (Hershberger, Schoenfeld, & Turkaspa, 2012).

Couples similar to Lisa and Jack, who might have been worried about PGD at the start, require multiple levels of support including baseline information and education of intricate and complex assisted reproductive and genetic information to understand the growing reproductive options. In regard to the Nash family, the nurses' primary concern was to give the parents appropriate information so that they could make the best decision for both Molly and Adam (Hershberger, Schoenfeld, & Turkaspa, 2012)..

Although nurses should support whatever the family's decision happens to be, they are still required to fulfill their professional obligation by addressing the initial ethical, legal and psychosocial concerns among high-genetic-risk couples surrounding PGD use. Foremost, couples may contemplate issues of eugenics regarding whether or not it is appropriate for parents to determine aspects of a future child's genetic composition (Kalfoglou, Scott, & Hudson,

2005). Couples may also be concerned about confidentiality and disclosure of genetic information to other family members, insurance companies and other payers and, at times, with themselves. Nurses should suggest visiting a counselor for further assistance. When the couple decides to move forward, as the Nash family did, nurses need to ensure that the couple is fully informed about the benefits and risks of such procedures (Adamson, 2010).

Conclusion

Undergoing genetic selection generally entails ethical concern, especially in cases such as the Nash family. In the Nash case, the children were not of age to consent to the terms the parents were suggesting, which brought into question child abuse. However, the genetically engineered embryo may have saved Molly Nash's life. With such extreme contrasts, families must consider the pros and cons to their individual situation, and make decisions that will benefit all participants. Nurses have the responsibility to teach their clients about all aspects of making decisions and provide support along the way. Nurses should be trustworthy, supportive sources, especially when the fates of innocent lives are at hand (Adamson, 2010).

References

Adamson GD. *Ethical considerations in genetic diagnosis and screening of embryos.* SRM: Sexuality, Reproduction, & Menopause. 2010;8(1):21–25.

Frankenfield, G. (2000). *The Nash family: Breaking new ground in medicine.* Retrieved from http://www.webmd.com/news/20001004/nash-family-breaking-new-ground-in-medicine

Hershberger, P., Schoenfeld, C., & Turkaspa, i. (2012). *Unraveling Preimplantation Genetic Diagnosis for High-Risk Couples Implications for Nurses at the Front Line of Care*. NCBI. Retrieved April 6, 2013, from US National Library of Medicine National Institutes of Health Search termSearch database (PMCID: PMC3408233 NIHMSID: NIHMS392986).

http://www.ncbi.nlm.nih.gov/pmc/articles/PMC3408233/

Kalfoglou AL, Scott J, Hudson K. *PGD patients' and providers' attitudes to the use and regulation of preimplantation genetic diagnosis*. Reproductive Biomedicine Online.2005;11(4):486–496. doi: 10.1016/S1472-6483(10)61145-5. [PubMed] [Cross Ref]

Simoncelli, T. (2003). *Pre-implantation genetic diagnosis: Ethical guidelines for responsible regulation*. International Center for Technology Assessment. Retrieved from *www.andrewkimbrell.org/doc/pgd%20guidelines.pdf*

Grading Rubric

Grading Criteria	Comments	Points
Paper		

• Introduction
  Nature & Scope of the case issue (a minimum of one source from the literature must be utilized in this discussion)
  10 points		

• Pro Perspective 10 points		
• Con Perspective 10 points		
• Nursing Responsibilities 10 points		
• Conclusion 5 points		
• Grammar/Spelling/Length 5 points		
• APA Format 5 points		
Pp Slides		
• Project information is summarized within the 10 slide limit established 10 points		
• Aesthetics of slide presentation are professional and allow for comfortable viewing on computer screen 10 points		
• Content of presentation is organized and flows logically to describe case study 10 points		
Discussion Board		
• Posted comments *to* peer groups 4 points		
• Replied to responses *from* peers 1 point		
Peer Evaluation 10 points		
Final Grade		/100

Rebecca Parker

www.ingramcontent.com/pod-product-compliance
Lightning Source LLC
Chambersburg PA
CBHW050045230526
45470CB00004B/1410